Difficult Patients

Senior commissioning editor: Mary Seager
Editorial assistant: Caroline Savage
Production controller: Anthony Read
Desk editor: Angela Davies
Cover designer: Helen Brockway

Difficult Patients

Joy Duxbury

BSc(Hons) RNT RMN RGN
Senior Lecturer in Health Studies,
Bolton Institute,
Bolton,
UK

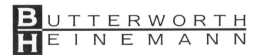

OXFORD   AUCKLAND   BOSTON   JOHANNESBURG   MELBOURNE   NEW DELHI

Butterworth-Heinemann
Linacre House, Jordan Hill, Oxford OX2 8DP
225 Wildwood Avenue, Woburn, MA 01801-2041
A division of Reed Educational and Professional Publishing Ltd

A member of the Reed Elsevier plc group

First published 2000

© Reed Educational and Professional Publishing Ltd 2000

British Library Cataloguing in Publication Data
Duxbury, Joy
    Difficult patients
    1. Nurse and patient   2. Patients – Psychology
    I. Title
    610.7'30699

    ISBN 0 7506 3838 9

Library of Congress Cataloguing in Publication Data
A catalogue record for this book is available from the Library of Congress

ISBN 0 7506 3838 9

Composition by Scribe Design, Gillingham, Kent
Printed and bound in Great Britain by Biddles Ltd, Guildford and
King's Lynn

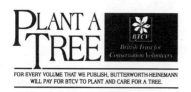

Contents

Introduction

Human interaction can be full of complexities and difficult situations, yet it is generally recognized that we live and work by a set of communication rules (Argyle, 1990). These range from the niceties of that first hello to the more complex relationship behaviours. Nursing is no different and can bring out the worst and the very best of human relationships. One of the greatest challenges a nurse can face is to encounter what he or she perceives to be a 'difficult patient' or, at least, a difficult situation based on needs, problems, personalities and past experience. To address this issue, having first both recognized and admitted that 'difficult patients' do indeed exist, a thread of what I can only describe as common sense prevails and is utilized throughout this book. This common sense underpins the ongoing guidelines offered when dealing with and ultimately 'caring' for a 'difficult' or potentially 'difficult' patient or client.

The terms 'patient' and 'client' will be used interchangeably throughout, given the many facets of health care and nursing roles that increasingly exist today. While nurses at every level, qualified and unqualified, and at every level of training, are the focus of discussions and guidelines offered, health care professionals generally may benefit from this approach. There are no exemptions from the need to enhance effective communication with patients whatever the setting, stage, or level of care involved.

Within the realms of social science and nursing, every situation, encounter and individual has the potential to be 'difficult'. For instance, the ward environment, the outpatients' department, the GP's surgery, and the community crisis centre are all potential minefields of emotion, uncertainty, physical or psychological disruption and vulnerability. As such, the crucial seeds of basic communication are paramount. A mixture of influences has shaped my approach to this text and the strategies and approaches offered. Undoubtedly, the world of psychology and counselling has been influential, particularly the works of both Gerard Egan and John Heron and their own individual models of helping. Exploration and application of these two approaches has been most useful in providing what I believe to be an integrated approach to therapeutic communication in the nurse–patient relationship. However, source material and inspiration has not stopped there. A wealth of personal experience, good and bad, has proved invaluable, as indeed has exploration of the increasing amount of literature examining human potential. A set of principles referred to simply as the rules are advocated in addition in an adapted form (Fein and Schneider, 1995) and, while criticized by some, have influenced my work. The incorporation of a variety of sources, in summary, has led to the development of a therapeutic set of rules, which are offered in the final stages of this book. These can be used not only as a reminder and summary of the key principles addressed but also as a springboard for care and standards of good practice in the nurse–patient relationship.

It is not my intention to provide or even attempt to provide a definitive research-based book on communication. There is endless material the reader can explore if wishing to pursue the same. It is, however, my intent to provide a compact approach to communicating with 'difficult patients' in the health care setting and, above all, to strive to provide an approach for all effective communication with patients. The underlying message being that we must make therapeutic communication a way of life for ourselves in both our professional and, if sought, personal roles. It is difficult and less effective to separate the two. In integrating therapeutic communication strategies as an overall approach to enhance all nursing care, relationships can be nurtured and potential problems that may precipitate the 'difficult patient' syndrome recognized. Prevention is the better approach and therapeutic communication is not only to be employed when difficulties in practice or 'difficult patients' are encountered. 'Difficult patients' may evolve in situations that appear to be out of our professional control and as such require very specific interventions for very specific needs, circumstances or individuals.

Chapter 1

The 'difficult patient'

The existence of the 'difficult patient': myth or reality?

The term, 'difficult patient' is not new to nursing and has continued to receive attention in various forms since the 1950s (Stockwell, 1984). Most professions face similar problems and many are familiar with the concept of the difficult customer. However, for nurses to acknowledge that 'difficult patients' do indeed exist is paramount, although emotive and problematic. Nurses are seen to be caring, compassionate and, above all, nurturing. They are expected by the public to be there for the frail, vulnerable and infirm 24 hours a day, unconditionally. To believe that there are some patients who are less likeable, more difficult and troublesome to care for, is an uncomfortable concept (Stockwell, 1984); yet, both nurses and patients alike know that such individuals do indeed exist. This becomes increasingly apparent as we continue to witness rising intolerance, greater impatience and growing expectations from patients (Rogers *et al.*, 1993; Department of Health, 1998).

If one accepts that difficult patients do exist, then the question of identity, location, number and cause needs to be addressed. When researching this book, stories from nurses about difficult patients were numerous. It seems they come in all shapes and sizes, inhabit every corner of the hospital domain and beyond, can be found in every nurse's collection of anecdotes and can have a whole host of reasons why they appear to be the difficult, often unlikeable, individuals they are. To reveal thoughts and feelings about difficult patients does not mean necessarily that we do not care or that we are not 'good nurses'. It does mean, however, that some patients do struggle to communicate effectively and, as such, need additional support. It also means that nurses must be encouraged to recognize the two-way process of communication (Kagan and Evans, 1995) and be aware of when they too may need help in communicating effectively. After all, there are undoubtedly 'difficult nurses', but that's another book entirely!

Numerous texts exist on the subject of communication, often covering a whole range of issues, albeit indirectly, concerning 'difficult patients'; for example, violence and aggression, non-compliance, expressions of pain, fear and anxiety, reluctant collaboration (Luker and Waterworth, 1990), social and individual psychology, sleep difficulties and specific patient problems that may result in difficult communication and the resulting 'patient labelling' that often occurs. This may include familiar labels such as 'the psychiatric patient' or others relating to ethnic minority groups, religion, sexuality or just plain individual choice (Stockwell, 1984).

Noticeably, there are certain issues that have received limited attention due to their delicate nature, in particular the 'difficult patient' and nurse relationship. It seems this is where an appropriate text is both lacking and long overdue. For instance a resource that recognizes problems and offers strategies for therapeutic practice in a succinct and accessible form; a manual of 'good practice' if you will, in the care and management of 'difficult patients' with commonly encountered and very specific needs.

In order to achieve such an approach it is my intention to adopt a two-tier format within this book. The first part offers an outline and discussion surrounding various theories and thoughts, enabling readers at all levels to gain insight into issues that surround problems in the nurse–patient relationship. The second part focuses upon practical frameworks which may guide the practitioner in his or her encounters with 'difficult patients'.

A wealth of information both personal and otherwise is drawn upon. No one difficult patient will be like another in how they present, why they present or in their response to nursing approaches. The experience of the individual is entirely unique. If answers were truly straightforward this book would have been written long ago or would not be necessary at all. The key is finding common ground and experiences that present in a collection of 'difficult patient' encounters and exploring potential communication strategies that may assist the nurse in his or her therapeutic response. This response, in turn, will lay the foundation for the development of a therapeutic relationship and the rewards that such a bond may reap. Such relationships may not only apply to the nurse–patient partnership, but may prove useful to all health care workers in their relationships, both private and professional. There are difficult individuals in all walks of life and the potential to be difficult lurks within us all.

Overall, it is anticipated that this book will provide the reader with the rules necessary for effective therapeutic relationships, particularly with difficult patients who have crossed the boundaries of acceptable behaviour given the context they are in. The practitioner's utilization of these rules will determine the success of interventions. Feedback and ongoing evaluation of performance in the nurse–patient relationship is crucial to the nurse following the rules and in selection of the best tools for the situation and individuals involved. If the chosen response does not work for one patient then there will be others to use and adapt. You will quickly learn as you follow the guidelines offered that the art of listening, observation, receptivity and adaptability are crucial skills when working with 'difficult patients'. This is not an easy task as the difficult client will often not recognize that they are being difficult or refuse to admit it. Any confrontation may, therefore, lead to an increase in the difficult behaviour presented or give way to a whole new range of problematic displays of maladaptive coping mechanisms.

The range of rules and tools identified throughout this book draw heavily upon the works of John Heron (1990), Richard Miller (1990), Nelson-Jones (1993), Fein and Schneider (1995) and Gerard Egan (1998) and reflect the personal approach and beliefs of the author. Rules are identified that can apply to all situations irrespective of behaviours encountered, problems expressed, individual patient or nurse involved. The rules serve as a 'way of being' (Rogers, 1980) and are meant to be used proactively. A range of strategies and communication tools are also identified throughout the main stream of the text and are based upon 'difficult patient types' and are mostly reactive. The skills necessary to utilize these tools successfully are examined in addition and complete the overall combined approach advocated for therapeutic communication.

Having outlined the format of this book, the 'difficult patient' is next examined in greater detail. While recognized as a real problem by a range of practitioners (Hadfield-Law, 1998), little is known about such patients. A range of behaviours has been examined in isolation, however, for instance, aggression (Wykes, 1994), non-compliance (Cameron, 1996), withdrawal, interference and so forth. Nurses encounter such patients on a regular basis. Behaviours such as these commonly result in difficulties either in the way they make us feel, or in the way they restrict the progress of our intended role. In some cases both. Hence, patients exhibiting these behaviours are perceived as difficult.

Most nurses at some point in their career have encountered such patients and experienced the sigh of relief when a particular individual has been discharged or referred on elsewhere to become somebody else's 'difficulty' or problem. Patients by the nature of their need to be admitted to hospital or referred in some way obviously have difficulties of some sort, yet not all patients become or earn the label of being difficult.

It was in the late 1950s when possible flaws in the nurse–patient relationship and communication difficulties were first identified as a concern. Stockwell (1984) focused upon the existence of 'unpopular patients' and met with animosity in general from the nursing profession. Today in the 1990s, journals are filled with material relating to therapeutic communication in nursing. An array of terms has emerged in response and include helping models (Heron, 1990; Egan, 1998), interpersonal skills (Kagan and Evans, 1995), interviewing skills (Newell, 1994), counselling and helping skills (Nelson Jones, 1991; Tschudin, 1993) and therapeutic communication (Arnold and Boggs, 1995). Irrespective of this, inadequacies prevail (Champken-Woods, 1992).

The view that there exist 'difficult patients' as opposed to 'unpopular patients' may be a less negative one. While it is increasingly accepted that there are patients who are problematic (Hadfield-Law, 1998), there is not the general assumption that such individuals are naturally disliked as a result. This does not mean that this may not be the case. Often when we experience difficult encounters with others there is a natural instinct to feel less drawn to them when compared to those who make us feel good (Smith and Hart, 1994). However, the portrayal of 'difficult patients' reflects concern regarding communication barriers or breakdown in effective communication. The emphasis is upon communication as a two-way process (Ellis *et al.*, 1995). It is, therefore, important not to lay sole blame upon patients, expecting change from them alone, but instead to examine the relationship (DOH, 1998). Those patients perceived by nurses to be 'difficult' and perception is a crucial issue, often need additional nursing time and assistance with the problems they face.

The focus of this book is the underlying principles of therapeutic communication and the promotion of more fruitful nurse–patient relationships, particularly those that are difficult. Prevention of an increase in patients who become 'difficult' for a variety of reasons is the emphasis. However, it is recognized that some factors may be out of nursing control. There will always be some situations and areas of need that fall outside the nursing remit and, as such, these will not be addressed in this book. However, my aim is to address that which is both within the control of the nurse in terms of personal behaviour and that which is realistically manageable within the nurse–patient relationship.

Difficult patients will mean different things to different people. Nurses may not always identify the same 'difficult patients' on their wards, units or caseloads, although there may be similar responses. Labels once applied can often spread. Unpopular patients in the past have tended to fall into certain categories of individual or type of problem (Ingles, 1961; Stockwell, 1984).

Difficult patients are often identified as individuals presenting behaviours which create barriers to effective nursing. If behaviour is the presenting problem, then largely, this means that nurses have the potential to be more effective in both understanding that behaviour and promoting more adaptive communications. If we solely take a dislike to a patient and refuse to explore the issues underlying our dislike for them, then they will be perceived as an unpopular patient as opposed to a difficult one and our care will be affected accordingly. Stockwell (1984) sought to examine the behaviour of nurses in response to unpopular patients, but no attempt was made to enhance nurse–patient relationships, although this was inherently recognized as a need throughout her book. It is my hope, however, that in this book the interdependency of the nurse–patient relationship be discussed. A range of strategies are presented to enhance communication with difficult patients in hospital and in the broader context.

Who is the 'difficult patient'?

Difficult patients are those who make us feel frustrated, uncomfortable or ineffective as nurses (Miller, 1990). Feeling uncomfortable may be the result of dislike for a patient or their behaviour, feeling frustrated at their progress, feeling unsure of their behaviour or how it makes us feel, or as a result of uncertainty about how to intervene. All of these things, in turn, may make us feel ineffective as nurses and unhappy with ourselves. We all by and large like to be liked and to feel useful. Given that nursing continues to be vocational in part, job satisfaction is all-important. Caring and being productive is a part of that job satisfaction and considered to be inherent in our role (Rodwell, 1996).

To repeatedly face difficult patients with whom we feel ill equipped or ill prepared to help can be demotivating.

The difficult patient is often the one who is most time consuming, even when ignored or avoided (Smith and Hart, 1994). In Stockwell's (1984) research, nursing staff clearly identified both popular and unpopular individuals and the apparent reasons for patients being classified as such. Nurses' attitudes towards unpopular patients were based on assumptions made about four main areas:

1. Personality factors – for instance bad tempered and selfish patients.
2. Communication factors – this included patients who were uncooperative or grumbling.
3. Nursing factors – such as feelings that this patient 'does not need to be in hospital'.
4. Attitude factors – for example, patients who are unwilling to accept treatment or who are reluctant to go home.

Personality and communication factors rated high overall in the determination of both 'popular' and 'unpopular' individuals. The patients whom the nurses indicated they least enjoyed looking after fell into two main groups. (1) Those who indicated in some way that they were not happy to be on the ward or with what was being done to or for them. This involved patients who grumbled, complained, or demanded attention. (2) Those whom the nursing staff felt did not need to be in hospital or in a particular ward setting. This was particularly the case for patients whose behaviour or communication difficulties did not outweigh perceived problems. This group included psychiatric patients, violent patients and patients from ethnic minorities (Stockwell, 1984). Previous studies have reflected similar qualities in those termed as 'bad patients' (Ritvo, 1963), but has also included the over-dependent, lazy, dishevelled (Highley and Norris, 1957), non-appreciative (Ritvo, 1963), overly emotional, immature, non-conforming (Schwartz, 1958; Ingles, 1961), and overly questioning (MacGregor, 1960). Patients who question practitioners are more commonly experienced today and often encouraged (Ashworth *et al.*, 1992; Department of Health, 1998).

Peterson (1967) argues 'a difficult patient is described as demanding, uncooperative, unresponsive to treatment, unappreciative or generally unlikeable. Actually a difficult patient is often one whose needs are not met – either emotionally or physically'. By definition it would appear it is this lack of attention to needs that may be the key to identifying the difficult patient who may have valid reasons for his or her behaviour. Miller (1990) argues that one person will find another difficult for one of three reasons:

- Because of threatening behaviour, actual or anticipated.
- Competitive behaviour, which includes specifically needing and seeking the attention of a nurse who may be focusing upon others. Jealousy may play a large part in this behaviour.
- And finally, stressful behaviour, whereby the individual feels he or she is being threatened.

Miller (1990) stresses that there are five ways in which one can portray the need to be difficult: they include behaviours expressing withdrawal, passivity, manipulation, aggression or violence. The latter two categories are increasingly problematic in today's health care settings (Health Service Advisory Committee, 1987; Wykes, 1994), particularly in contrast to recent years. Each category can be defined in the following way:

1. Withdrawal, which is defined as the act of refusing to interact.
2. Passivity, which involves failure to take any action. Non-compliance is often a feature of both withdrawal and passivity.
3. Manipulation, meaning to practise the use of devious and dishonest means.
4. Aggression, which is the expression of anger with an implication of violence. Confrontation is included in this category.
5. Violence, which is defined as a physical act against others, self or property, which is intended to or does cause damage.

Combined, these five categories of behaviour appear to cover the wealth of possible communication difficulties a nurse can encounter when presented with a 'difficult client'. The actual complexities of presenting behaviours are not so simple, however, and can often be more complicated. Irrespective of this, Miller's (1990) delineation of difficulties is a useful one in which to explore the behaviours of clients who are perceived as problematic and the possible solutions advocated.

Difficult patients are difficult people and it therefore seems useful to examine in the first instance the nature of a difficult person. Cava (1996) suggests a difficult person is one whose behaviour causes difficulties for you and for others. Dealing with difficult people simply means dealing with difficult behaviour. Therefore, behaviour needs to be addressed. Effective communication has little to do with liking or disliking a patient, although this will always contribute in some way, but more to do with recognizing behaviour that appears to be difficult, understanding it in its context and using effective strategies to deal with it. Communication, as mentioned previously, is a two-way process (Hartley, 1993). You react to the patient who, in turn, reacts to you. If this reaction is negative, a vicious circle ensues. We may not be able to directly control other people's behaviour and nor should we endeavour to do so, but by learning how to manage our own behaviour and developing appropriate techniques, we can learn to influence others in a more positive and constructive way (Cava, 1996). It is about learning how to manage and take responsibility for your side of the two-way transaction.

Difficult patients, if we let them, can affect us in the following ways. They can:

- Make us lose our cool.
- Force us, to some extent, to react in ways we are not happy with.
- Prevent us from doing our job effectively.
- Manipulate us and use underhanded methods to get their own way or meet their immediate needs.
- Make us feel guilty.
- Make us anxious, upset, frustrated, angry, inferior, defeated or experience other negative feelings.
- Make us do their share of the work particularly while they remain passive (Cava, 1996).

Or can they?

Too often we let others affect how we perceive or feel about ourselves. In order to tackle difficult patients successfully, it is essential that as nurses we are self-aware and have a degree of self-control. This is all-important. Commonly and often without realizing, our actions can contribute to difficult behaviour in others. For instance, there may be times when we encourage patients to be passive and overly dependent (Brearley, 1990) or non-compliant, non-conforming and ill-informed (Cameron, 1996). In order to reduce such behaviours, strategies to promote negotiation and participation are advocated (Ashworth *et al.*, 1992). Facilitation is crucial if these strategies are to be successful, and include information giving, enabling and supportive skills (Heron, 1990). Before greater cooperation and communication can be encouraged, first, better understanding of the specific needs of individuals according to their presenting difficult behaviour must be identified. Below is a more detailed examination of the most commonly encountered difficult behaviours that may be exhibited by patients (Miller, 1990).

Ways of being difficult

1 *The act of withdrawal.* This, suggests Miller (1990), is the act of refusing to interact or to cooperate due to disinterest, denial, fear, protest, refusal on moral grounds or just plain laziness. Withdrawal may not be something a patient actively chooses to do or may, in fact, not be a conscious decision. Patients may become withdrawn, opt out of treatment or go as far as discharging themselves for a whole host of reasons. We all come in all shapes and sizes and each of us has a background of varying experience, both good and bad, that may influence our actions. Some of these experiences may be with the health service previously, while other patients may never have dealt with hospitals, hospitalization or consultations before.

Withdrawal may be the result of a whole array of real or potential physical problems such as pain, discomfort, lack of sleep, immobility and disorientation, or as a result of psychological factors including criticism, confusion, uncertainty, frustration, fear, anxiety or poor support. It may commonly involve a combination of the two. Withdrawal due to lack of cooperation can be most frustrating and seen as an act of rejection or dislike by the nurse. It may be that a patient is trying to come to terms with some bad news and unable to become involved in his or her own care due to fear, denial that anything is happening or a lack of input/information from the nurse as to how to progress. Assumptions are commonly made on initial contact about an individual's ability to retain and comprehend new information. These assumptions generally seem to be the most common culprit in precipitating difficult behaviour. For example assumptions that are often incorrect, over generalized, misconceived, non-person-centred or based on insufficient knowledge and understanding of the 'individual' (Miller, 1990).

When threatened, there are instinctively one of two options to take; to fight or to flight (Powell and Enright, 1993). In reality, there is the additional option to stay and communicate, even when faced with danger. However, our first response often without thought and based upon emotion, commonly involves the primitive behaviours of defence, attack or withdrawal. This is a crucial factor when nursing patients who are withdrawn or who appear to be isolated. The nurse is dealing with an individual who is experiencing threat, or their perception of it, and as such is making a choice to 'back off', and is often struggling to communicate effectively. Withdrawn patients as such have their own set of needs, not least of which is to identify what and how that threat is perceived by them. Only by understanding the patient's individual experience of hospitalization or distress can we ever begin to appreciate their behaviour in context, and develop the necessary principles of therapeutic communication.

In some instances, withdrawn patients are perceived by nurses in a positive light, particularly if they are those who make few demands upon nursing staff. Stockwell (1984) identified such patients as 'popular patients'. Withdrawal is viewed in a more negative light when it is seen to hinder or prevent progress or interfere with the successful implementation of nursing care. For instance, the client who is very quiet but cooperates by mobilizing when expected and adheres to a medication regimen is not seen as difficult. Alternatively, the female patient who is hostile in her silence and will not cooperate with treatment would commonly be perceived by nursing staff to be 'difficult' (Miller, 1990). Of the four categories of difficult behaviour identified by Miller (1990), each behaviour is interchangeable and may not be seen in isolation.

Assessment of patient behaviour and how it is interpreted will also be affected by the personalities of the people involved. Individual situations and past knowledge and experience of any given patient in addition may contribute. There may, indeed, be some circumstances in which it is both perfectly normal and acceptable not to interact with other people for a while and withdraw from direct communication. For example, having just received bad news postoperatively or when trying to rest or sleep. Behaviour is variable and may only be periodic. As such, withdrawal may be partial or intermittent and influenced by a variety of factors within the health care setting. These factors may include the nurse, time, events, atmosphere and environment, both physical and otherwise. Each of these issues must be taken into consideration when caring for the withdrawn patient.

2 *Passivity and the uncooperative patient.* Passivity is 'the failure to take action and is different from withdrawal in that a passive person is often willing to allow interactions to take place and, indeed, relies upon others involved in the interaction as a means of remaining in a passive state' (Miller, 1990). Passive patients, although viewed as difficult patients in some instances, may be a product of the health care system and may once have been valued

as ideal patients. They may be the result of a struggle to adjust to new ground rules such as greater collaboration care (Luker and Waterworth, 1990). On the one hand they may be patients who consciously or otherwise do not wish to take responsibility for their own condition or progress, while, on the other hand, may just be actively obstructive.

The biomedical model has commonly perpetuated passivity in patients (Walsh and Ford, 1992) but as efforts increase to move away from this approach, greater numbers of 'difficult clients' of the passive type may be identified. Abdication of responsibility in such individuals can be just as problematic for the nurse as the patient who will not comply with treatment or who prolongs their need for health care by not helping him- or herself. Patients in this group can also be perceived as 'demanding'. By prolonging the need for nursing and medical attention and delaying a return to well-being, greater nursing attention is required which, in turn, is additional strain on already limited resources. This does not help to reduce the increasing nursing workload and, as such, may make these clients particularly unpopular and difficult to nurse. Stockwell (1984) found such patients to be subtly demanding attention in a more acceptable form.

Whatever the underlying impetus, the result is the same. Others find themselves making decisions and taking action for the passive person. For years, the nurse–patient and doctor–patient relationship has been based on foundations of passivity. It is hardly surprising therefore, that what we witness in the passive patient may be the result of someone who is struggling to adjust to new objectives. It is, therefore, at least initially, the responsibility of the nurse to ensure that roles are redefined and identified clearly to patients. This sets the scene for negotiation and participation as opposed to passivity and control.

Passive patients will not always be deemed to be 'difficult' and there are clearly various shades of passivity. 'There may be occasions when it is best to be passive as in a medical emergency when staff are more able to go about their business if the patient has a degree of passivity' (Miller, 1990). However, given the emphasis in present day health care to encourage greater independence in clients, prolonged passivity can be problematic (Brearley, 1990). 'Independence and passivity are not compatible' (Miller, 1990).

3 *Manipulation and defensiveness – challenging behaviour.* Manipulation is defined as using devious and dishonest means to affect another's behaviour or achieve an anticipated outcome (Miller, 1990). The difficult patients most commonly identified in

this group by nurses are those who display 'demanding' or 'attention seeking' behaviour. I prefer to use the term 'attention needing', which reflects a basic underlying need. It also changes how we might view these patients. Demanding patients may be perceived in a variety of ways. For instance, they may be:

- noisy
- complaining
- 'clingy'
- overly emotional
- grumpy
- or generally, dissatisfied.

The attention needing displays that then result may include any one or several of the following behaviours:

- Feigning illness or discomfort in order to prolong hospitalization or care
- Making seemingly unsubstantiated complaints or playing one nurse off against another
- Seeking constant attention that does not reflect the patient's actual level of need, believed or otherwise.

The need for attention from staff is important in its own right for some patients and the resulting possession of such attention from nurses has a value all of its own. The problem leading to hospitalization may be secondary. Patients who seem to need what nurses perceive as unrealistic levels of constant nursing attention (and this in itself must be taken into account), do indeed have needs that ultimately must be addressed. Miller's (1990) use of the term manipulation is possibly inappropriate in a health care context, although some nurses, I know, would argue otherwise. While it may not be a term consciously overused in nursing, it is one frequently referred to when describing troublesome patients who are demanding or attention needing. In many respects most patients are demanding in one form or another, purely by the nature of their lack of well-being and need for medical/nursing attention.

Every patient presents their own set of individual needs and problems. So what is it particularly that makes us think that one patient is more demanding than another? And when and how do we decide that a certain level of being demanding is too much and, therefore, determined to be 'attention seeking' as opposed to an acceptable need for nursing attention? This is by no means an easy issue and a whole host of forces are at play in this decision making process. The following factors may contribute to this process:

1. Personality. The personalities of the individuals involved (nurse and patient). We identify with some patients and as a result are far more accepting of them, making many more allowances than we would for others. The introverted nurse who finds the extrovert patient very loud and interfering highlights this. An extrovert nurse may perceive such a patient in a very different way and warm to their outgoing nature. As nurses, we have to adjust to the individual personalities of all our patients but, inevitably, some we will like instinctively more than others. We are only human. The label 'difficult patient' tends to be a negative one and as such will be more readily attached to those we find more difficult to like.
2. Type of patient problem, which leads to difficult communication. Issues related to 'type' and race of patient appear to colour our judgement as identified by Stockwell (1984). For example, psychiatric patients and patients who find it difficult to communicate, such as those who cannot speak English, are frequently labelled 'unpopular'. This may be the result of lack of knowledge about individuals with certain problems, frustration at feeling helpless, uncertainty about how to communicate effectively or collective socialization which determines 'good' and 'bad' patients.
3. Group conformity. The issue of collective socialization in nursing warrants some discussion within itself. Having had 17 years of experience in nursing, in various specialities and from both the nurse and patient side of the bed, it becomes apparent that nurses have the ability to group together in their dissatisfaction and avoidance of certain patients. This may purely be a view that is passed on from one nurse to another during handovers, while giving care or at team meetings. It is far more acceptable for a team of nurses to come to the conclusion that a patient is 'difficult' as responsibility is diffused. As a result no one individual can be accused of being uncaring (Shulka, 1988). There is also less likely to be a sense of failure among individual nurses if all the nurses in one team agree that this problem patient is just too difficult to nurse or help. This diffusion of responsibility is commonly seen in team nursing (Shulka, 1988).
4. Past experience. Past experience may very much influence a nurse's judgement in identifying any one individual as 'difficult'. Having had an uncomfortable experience with one patient who can be easily categorized may, in turn, colour one's view of similar patients, even before we have had the opportunity to get to know them.

Whatever the combination of factors that influence perceptions of who is demanding and who is not, in response there is a tendency to feel uncomfortable. Possible reasons for this are as follows:

- They require too much nursing time or frustrate us because we cannot give the time necessary.
- They make us feel uncomfortable because they appear intrusive and overstep the boundaries we clearly lay for the nurse–patient relationship.
- We do not like the way such patients make us feel about ourselves or about our ability to be effective nurses. Of course nobody can truly make us feel a certain way, we choose to react as we do. However, realistically, we are indeed influenced by the actions of others.

Overall, the main problem with manipulative behaviour or our identification of it, is that it is undoubtedly stressful and can distract the attention of the nurse from the patient's real problem(s) (Miller, 1990). Nurses tend to avoid patients who make excessive demands and become afraid that when they encounter the patient again, a new or additional demand will be made. As a result, there is often an increase in 'detachment' or gradual withdrawal (Smith and Hart, 1994). This, in turn, may make the patient more needy and more demanding and a vicious circle emerges.

'Demanding' patients pose particular problems to health care professionals in that they present a degree of threat. Many nurses in the process of avoidance, withdrawal or detachment know realistically that they are failing to communicate therapeutically (Smith and Hart, 1994). As a result they know that they too may face the hostility of detachment, dislike, withdrawal and ultimately anger and/or confrontation. Demanding patients are indeed possibly perceived as a threat in the first place for this very reason; that they can reject us or harm us in some way or most certainly enhance any feeling of inadequacy, professional or otherwise.

Effective communication is, largely, about honesty. We may be dishonest if we fail to address a problem with our clients in order to avoid discomfort ourselves. Most patients crave the opportunity to talk and be listened to (Arnold and Boggs, 1995). All patients have a story to tell and the process of making patients feel worthwhile and valued begins with giving time and listening accurately to what is being said (and in many instances what is not) (Egan, 1998). If manipulation is to be defined as the deliberate act of using dishonest and devious means (Miller, 1990), then to attach this label to patients does little to inspire more fruitful nurse–patient relationships. Manipulation is premeditated dishonesty and it is unrealistic to believe that all 'demanding' patients are sat plotting ways to make the nurse's job a difficult one. It is true to say, however, that some individuals need more support and ongoing reassurance than others and it is possibly when such basic needs are not being met that the 'difficult' behaviour results. Often the process of explanation and negotiation can be crucial in preventing the escalation of demanding and later 'attention seeking' behaviour. Such behaviour if unattended to may progress to maladaptive forms of communication including feigning illness, refusing to cooperate, preventing recovery, extreme displays of emotion such as anger and aggression or making demands that may appear unreasonable and obstructive (Miller, 1990). In keeping with the positive emphasis of this book and the promotion of nurse–patient relationships, the term attention seeking patients shall be replaced with the more productive term 'attention needing patients'. To need as opposed to actively seek, provides a whole new emphasis on which to base future encounters with challenging patients and shall be addressed in more detail later in this text.

4 *Confrontation and aggression.* Aggression and violence are on the increase in health care (Health Service Advisory Committee, 1987; Royal College of Psychiatrists, 1998) which presents the nurse, in particular, with a range of problems. Both behaviours are a direct threat to safety and as such are the most feared form of confrontation both anticipated and/or experienced by nurses across specialities. It has been reported that nurses in certain specialities or nursing environments are more prone to attack or threat of attack than others (Health Service Advisory Committee, 1987). While it may be true that areas including Accident and Emergency departments, the community and mental health settings have a more widely reported incidence of aggression (Health Service Advisory Committee, 1987), all nurses are increasingly at risk. Many nurses report episodes of patient anger on a regular basis that may or may not then escalate into something more violent (Duxbury, 1999a). Irrespective of place of work, nurses on a daily basis face confrontation from patients and their kin (Poster and Ryan, 1993). This confrontation can take on many forms and is often precipitated by a combination of factors including any number of the following:

- Growing expectations from patients.
- Stretched resources.
- Increased waiting times.

- Low staff morale.
- Pressure of work.
- Cutbacks
- Lowered tolerance generally.
- Rising stress levels in both nurses and patients, which in turn affects tolerance levels.
- Impaired communication as a result of all of the above.

The health care sector can be a minefield of anxieties, complaints, fears and frustrations, which will inevitably result in confrontation if not recognized and addressed. When dealing with 'difficult patients' of the confrontational kind, this lack of recognition is both largely the problem and the solution. The need to communicate effectively and to both recognize and address the difficulties of being a patient, is paramount.

Hospitals by the nature of their environment and patients by the nature of their needs provide a highly emotive atmosphere. Confrontation, therefore, can manifest in many forms and may commonly include complaints, anger, aggression and ultimately violence. It may also include hostile or non-hostile enquiries that confront the nurse with frequently difficult and uncomfortable dilemmas. For instance, questions regarding prognosis, requests for additional information about care and treatment and even questions related to the nurse's knowledge, skill, ability and suitability. Patients are far more assertive and aware of their rights than ever before (Department of Health, 1991). However, the role of negotiator and patient advocate in nursing is relatively new and one with which the nurse is still to some extent struggling to adjust (Brearley, 1990; Ashworth *et al.*, 1992; Gates, 1994).

The confrontational patient poses a range of both real and potential problems for the nurse. The biggest problem is the degree of threat involved. The words aggression and assertion are frequently misinterpreted by patients when upset and can lead to similar displays of difficult behaviour.

'Assertion refers to the ability to express one's views in a clear, confident, direct manner, without denying the rights of another. By implication, an aggressive manner, therefore, fails to acknowledge one's own rights' (Farrell and Gray, 1992).

In an effective relationship assertive behaviour should be non-threatening; however, this can frequently be perceived as threatening by both nurses and patients. Adjustments in thinking are imperative and will influence perceptions of who is and who is not a 'difficult patient'. The assertive patient can be an ally as opposed to an enemy.

Farrell and Gray (1992) argue it is important to raise the subject of assertion for two reasons:

1. First, because by understanding the differences between assertion and aggression, we can recognize and accept that aggression should and need not be tolerated within the nurse–patient relationship.
2. Secondly, that assertion may be a useful tool for practitioners in response to certain aggressive situations and individuals. This will be dealt with more fully when exploring therapeutic responses to 'confrontational patients' in later sections.

A third important point relates to patient assertion, which can be very positive. By encouraging patients to express their views and perspectives in a mature way, greater understanding of their needs can be facilitated. Hence the growth of health psychology in the last decade (Ogden, 1998).

Aggression, on the other hand, is the expression of anger with an implication of violence. Violence is the actual physical act against another, self or property, which is intended inevitably to cause damage (Miller, 1990). This may be physical or psychological. The anticipation of aggressive behaviour, which includes fear of the unknown and of possible escalation, can be just as intimidating (if not more so) as the actual physical act of violence. The threat of violence is often imminent with the expression of anger or other aggressive behaviour. Commonly, it is not simply enough to feel an emotion, there is also the urge to express it in some form, which may or may not manifest in violence. Past experience will influence our concern over an aggressive encounter with a patient as will our confidence to be able to respond effectively. The latter is often a crucial part of our ability to defuse an aggressive outburst.

Although the confrontational patient is probably most greatly feared for his or her potential to become aggressive, verbally or physically, an array of confrontational behaviour from difficult patients is possible. This may include any of the following:

- Concern from patients about care received or not received. Complaints may be both informal and formal. The former often takes the form of general comments to one or many nurses, while the latter involves patients who formally lodge a complaint, verbal or written.
- A disagreement regarding a care approach which may then lead to non-compliance. For instance, refusal to take medication, to change lifestyle, to rest or pursue a recommended pathway of

treatment. Such confrontations over care are particularly common in the mental health arena or with patients with chronic, long-term problems who may see no need for given approaches or no immediate effect (Cameron, 1996).

- Patients who refuse to cooperate when their values do not conform to those of the medical profession. This may range from strong religious beliefs regarding various medical interventions or to lifestyle choices that may not facilitate a chosen nursing approach. For instance, a patient with cancer may not wish to pursue traditional medical approaches but may opt instead to follow a course of alternative therapy. Numerous health belief models encourage patients to express their opinions about care options and, hence, reject the view that such behaviour is confrontational (Ogden, 1998).
- Assertive patients who make both reasonable and acceptable demands by requesting information, response, high standards and support, yet who may still be perceived as a threat to nursing authority and ability to give care.
- Patients who display highly emotive behaviours such as fear, sadness, anxiety and need. Many nurses continue to find it difficult to cope with expressions of emotion be it their own or from the patients they care for (Burnard and Morrison, 1991).
- Aggressive and violent patients.
- Patients who overstep what is viewed as nurse–patient relationship boundaries.This may include patients who over self-disclose (in our minds at least), or look to extend the relationship beyond that of a professional one (Arnold and Boggs, 1995).
- Patients who interfere with the care of others and patients who are sexually intrusive or explicit.

Each of these examples present their own set of challenges for the nurse and may involve clients who are viewed as difficult or confrontational. No one set of behaviours is more problematic or distressing for the nurse than another. There is no hierarchy of difficult behaviour and nor should there be. It depends upon the individuals involved, the context and timing. As such, each will be rated and perceived by different nurses in different ways depending upon experience, personality, personal and professional resources, knowledge, confidence and moment in time. What may be perceived as a threat one day, may appear less troublesome in the light of a new day. Personal and contextual variables are undoubtedly all important in our experience of and with difficult patients. DeVito (1986) argues that a powerful mitigating factor in the production of what we class as difficult behaviour stems from the fact that most people like to be liked. Enhancement of self-esteem contributes to the establishment of any relationship. There is no reason why this should be any different in the nurse–patient relationship. The patient may develop a 'difficult persona' because he or she ultimately feels disliked or undervalued. The nurse may then respond in an equally hostile or defensive way (Smith and Hart, 1994), believing that the display of difficult behaviour from the patient is either a personal attack or a show of dislike for that nurse or group of nurses.

For many of us, in fact, the difficult behaviour and difficult patients we encounter are far from being life-threatening to either nurse or patient. Rather, say Farrell and Gray (1992), it is a threat only at the intrapersonal level. When we are 'told off' or spoken to harshly or rejected in some way, we react instinctively to protect ourselves. It would appear that, in some situations, saving face can be just as important as saving life (Farrell and Gray, 1992).

The old adage 'sticks and stones may break my bones but names will never hurt me', may bear some inaccuracies. Vulnerability and low resilience can affect us all. The most minor of slights from a difficult patient can have lasting effects both on how we feel about ourselves and how we relate to and perceive other patients in the future. Farrell and Gray (1992) advocate there are two very important messages here when faced with difficult patients of any sort:

1. First, as nurses we need to be able to recognize each difficult situation for what it is and look beyond any hurt we may be feeling initially, to the broader, more objective perspective of why this individual is displaying such behaviour. In this way we become less subjective.
2. Secondly, we need to be able to examine and enhance our interpersonal skills in relation to effective therapeutic communication. This naturally involves scrutinizing our own professional behaviour, including that which we are good at and that which we need to work on.

Protective versus uncooperative behaviour

In summary, the various displays of difficult behaviour one might encounter can be broadly placed into two distinct categories. They are patients who are noticeably perceived as being uncooperative via manipulation and confrontation, this I have termed *defensive behaviour*, and those who are more *self-protective*, including withdrawn and passive patients. The protective group incorporates patients who exhibit a general lack of cooperation, which may or may not be intentional. Difficult patients who are protective often present in a less hostile manner than those who are defensive and intent on being hostile by disrupting treatment or by posing a threat. While it can be problematic to pigeon hole all patients or their behaviours in such an objective way, or equally difficult to believe that some patients are intent on behaving in a threatening way, there will always exist a small minority of individuals who wish to inflict harm on their fellow humans, whomever they might be and whatever the setting.

Difficult patients themselves will also commonly experience a level of threat and discomfort. In many cases there may be a range of valid reasons why their behaviour has become difficult. This is an important point and addresses the issue that the existence of difficult patients is not only a concern for the patient and/or nurse in isolation, but a mutual responsibility that can only be addressed by joint exploration and negotiation. In order to be effective, one must be able to determine the level and degree of non-cooperation and how it translates in terms of behaviour and underlying motivation. Non-cooperation may be a deliberate act to block progress, a personal attack against an individual practitioner, a protective defence (conscious or otherwise), or a genuine lack of knowledge and awareness. Only when these issues are explored and determined can an effective therapeutic programme be initiated that will address the relevant needs of the individuals involved.

The most beneficial approach to ensuring that the needs of the 'difficult patient' are met is to focus on the positive challenge facing the nurse and the ultimate difference he or she can make. To view patients solely in a negative light can only do harm and perpetuate the 'difficult patient syndrome'. Instead, one must try to put subjectivity to one side and objectively seek to intervene, recognizing that the patient may be experiencing a degree of distress; for instance, fear, anxiety, uncertainty, frustration, anger or ignorance. Address the underlying distress and the feelings of the individual and cooperation may be more obtainable. Ignore or avoid the problem or individual and the difficulties will continue. Communication and lack of it works both ways. Nurses are accountable for patient well-being and any action that may promote or prevent possible progress of that well-being (United Kingdom Central Council for Nursing, Midwifery and Health Visiting, 1992).

While communication is widely recognized as a two-way process (Sundeen *et al.*, 1994), it is impossible for any individual, be they nurse or patient, not to communicate. Verbal and non-verbal messages and images of who we are, are communicated all the time. Patients, whomever they are, are vulnerable. Each new situation and experience in health care brings with it a new set of difficulties. A nurse with effective relationship-building skills and the will to listen actively can have a positive impact upon a patient's experience of trauma, irrespective of the difficulties he or she is facing. It is those patients with specific vulnerabilities who will pose a real challenge and continue to present as difficult patients.

Chapter 2

The basic skills of therapeutic communication

The exploration of communication skills in the health care setting is not a new concern. Countless terms have appeared for some time now and include counselling, interpersonal skills, interviewing skills, problem solving, helping skills and models and, not least of all, therapeutic communication. All appear to have their place within the nurse–patient relationship and are influenced and shaped by various nursing/helping models, the nursing process and a number of counselling frameworks. Many are inter-related in their objectives and are clearly defined, whilst others are blurred in definition.

The term 'therapeutic communication' applies most naturally to the nurse–patient relationships and translates as a goal-directed, focused dialogue between nurse and client that is specifically tailored to the needs of that client (Severtsen, 1990). Arnold and Boggs (1995) argue this process involves the exchange of ideas, feelings and attitudes related to desired health care outcomes; as such it is an unavoidably mutual affair, a complementary process in which all parties must be actively engaged (Arnold and Boggs, 1995). When this engagement fails in the therapeutic partnership and is not pursued by either patient or nurse, then communication problems can result which, in turn, can highlight problems associated with a difficult patient. This is an important aspect. It is only when we are open to the realization that communication is and must be a two-way process, that we can accept our part to play in the development, management and possible prevention of difficult patients.

Arnold and Boggs (1995) argue that effective therapeutic conversation is a lot like playing ball. To play successfully, the participants (in this case both patient and nurse) must be active players and pay careful attention to the ball in transit. Throwing and receiving the ball is not a random affair. The ball must be thrown in such a way that the receiver can easily catch it. Once caught, unless dropped, the ball is returned to the sender with a similar degree of accuracy and care. Some balls will inevitably miss their mark. As such the nurse must adopt a high degree of responsibility as both a sender and a receiver in judging the speed and journey of the ball and how it is returned. In the role of sender, giving a message requires careful accuracy if the receiver (patient) is to catch it. For instance, if the message is thrown too high and is beyond the patient's comprehension or too fast, the ball or message may not be understood. The nurse as receiver must then be prepared to watch for and catch the client's communication accurately via both verbal and non-verbal feedback. Although it is often taken for granted that this is a natural process for most people, this is not always the case. Once a message is received by the nurse, the most appropriate response and channel is adopted to send further messages (Arnold and Boggs, 1995). We, therefore, rely heavily upon all our senses and sources of information when making such interpretations. This, in turn, allows us to build an ongoing picture and may help us to understand the needs and specific problems of each patient and how best to respond. The primary difference between interpersonal and therapeutic communication is the emphasis upon both purpose and focus in the promotion of patient well-being, as such therapeutic communication lends itself well to helping models (Egan, 1998).

Health care professionals including nurses are currently under scrutiny and to some extent criticism regarding the effectiveness of their communication skills. Limitations have been found in the quality and quantity of nurse communication with patients (Davis and Fallowfield, 1994; Audit Commission, 1991), some of which are highlighted in the Spotlight on Research item below.

Spotlight on Research No. 1

Factors which influence how nurses communicate with cancer patients (Wilkinson, 1991)

A study which aimed to determine:
1. the extent to which nurses facilitate or block patients' communication;
2. whether there is a relationship between nurses' verbal behaviours and their levels of anxiety, social support, work support and attitude to death;
3. nurses' difficulties in caring.

continued

continued
Communication is one of the most important aspects of nursing. Evidence suggests that nurses experience communication difficulties and frequently block patients from divulging their worries or concerns. Findings reveal that, in particular, there is an overall poor level of facilitative communication.

Background

Most interactions with patients occur when physical tasks are carried out and physical tasks rather than psychological aspects of care appear to dominate most nurse–patient communication (Faulkner, 1985). Nurses themselves admit that communicating with cancer patients is difficult (Wilkinson, 1986), but the exact problems have not been identified. It is suggested that difficulties arise because nurses do not have the verbal skills to assess how patients feel about their illness or have the skills but just do not use them.

Methodology

Subjects Fifty four registered nurses were randomly selected from a specialist and non-specialist hospital. The mean age of the sample was 28 years, 37 nurses were single, 18 were married and a mix of religious backgrounds was noted. Nineteen nurses had attended a communication skills course of 1–14 days in length.

Design An analytical relational survey was used.

Method The subjects completed three audio-taped histories (one with a new cancer patient, a patient with a recurrence and a patient for palliative care), a self-administered questionnaire and a semi-structured audio-taped interview.

Results

The questionnaire results were analysed using SSPSX and the tape-recorded histories were transcribed and rated by one of two independent psychologists. Findings revealed that nurses could be categorized as facilitators, ignorers (those who ignored patients' emotional cues), informers (those that largely gave information) and mixers (those that used a mixture of both facilitative and blocking strategies). The majority of nurses relied upon blocking tactics to prevent patients from divulging their problems.

Conclusion

The findings of this study support previous studies on communication skills. Despite an increase in communication skills training today, nurses in this sample were limited communicators with cancer patients and found facilitation difficult.

Based on
Wilkinson, S. (1991) Factors which influence how nurses communicate with cancer patients. *Journal of Advanced Nursing*, **16**, 677–688.

A list of deficiencies in the communication skills of health professionals has been identified by Davis and Fallowfield (1994). These deficiencies range from lacking very basic personal and social skills to inadequacies in the more advanced skills necessary for therapeutic interventions. They are as follows:

1. Failure to greet patients appropriately, to introduce themselves or to explain their actions to patients.
2. Failure to elicit easily available information especially major worries and expectations.
3. Acceptance of imprecise information and the failure to seek clarification.
4. Failure to check the professional's understanding of the situation against the patient's.
5. Neglect of covert and overt cues provided verbally or otherwise by the patient.
6. Failure to encourage questions or to answer them appropriately.

7. Avoidance of information about the personal, family and social situations of patients including problems in these areas.
8. Failure to elicit information about the patient's feelings and perceptions of the illness experienced.
9. A directive style with closed questions predominating, frequent interruptions and failure to let the patient talk spontaneously.
10. Focusing too quickly without exploring information.
11. Failure to provide information adequately about diagnosis, treatment, side effects or prognosis, or to check subsequent understanding.
12. Failure to understand from the patient's viewpoint and hence to be effectively supportive (Cameron and Gregor 1987).
13. Poor use of reassurance.

This list is by no means exhaustive and is not solely based upon the observations of nurse–patient communication. However, the problem areas listed highlight crucial deficiencies in effective communication skills in many health care settings, and consequently serious weaknesses in the nurse–patient relationship. Practitioners must carry the greater responsibility for addressing some of these concerns.

It is not my intention to imply that all nurses communicate inadequately or, if they do, that they do so all of the time. We all have different strengths and weaknesses that may fluctuate in different situations. However, the evidence does seems to suggest that there are sufficiently large numbers of workers within health care environments who exhibit poor, reduced or impaired communication, to warrant greater attention to the development of therapeutic relationships (Davis and Fallowfield, 1994). Such deficiencies can lead to dissatisfaction for both nurse and patient. For instance, inaccurate or impaired diagnosis and understanding (this is closely linked to inadequate empathy skills), problems with compliance, impaired recovery rates, and a lack of self-reliance may contribute to decreased patient autonomy (Davis and Fallowfield, 1994). Closer examination of these problems soon reveals behaviours that are closely associated with the range of 'difficult patients' identified earlier in the book; for example, passivity, withdrawal, manipulation and anger. These are uncooperative and at times defensive behaviours.

Reasons for such a breakdown in the utilization of effective therapeutic communication and associated strategies, incorporate a complex mixture of increasingly outdated factors. These include:

• An overly prescribed to and widely accepted medical ethos.

- The use of power by health care workers for protection and self-preservation.
- The perpetuated 'expert model' that subtly advocates that nurses control decision making due to an imbalance of knowledge and so power.
- A lack of identified frameworks and policies that lend themselves to effective and therapeutic communication.
- A nurse-led service as opposed to a patient-led approach (this is slowly changing).
- A general lack of substantial training and development in therapeutic communication (Davis and Fallowfield, 1994).

The adverse effects of poor communication with patients may last for a long time. This is particularly so in health care settings when people are ill and, therefore, more vulnerable, isolated and facing difficult situations in unfamiliar surroundings.

Having seen how communication failures can exacerbate problematic behaviour in certain vulnerable patients, let us now explore some of the crucial ingredients necessary to enhance therapeutic communication and the frameworks that can facilitate this development. The two helping models chosen to promote awareness and skills when caring for difficult patients are those of Gerard Egan (1998) and John Heron's Six Category Intervention Analysis Framework (Heron, 1990). Both have a tremendous amount to offer the nurse if used selectively and with an understanding of what one is trying to achieve.

This chapter is an introduction to these two models and the guidance each can offer. This guidance includes both the general principles of therapeutic communication and the more specific strategies needed to care for the various types of difficult patient. It is only on greater examination of these two frameworks that the strategies advocated can be truly appreciated and become a way of communicating in reality and practice. They will change not only your professional interactions for the better but also your personal ones if practised and rehearsed at every opportunity. As such it is imperative that when analysing your own behaviour in dealing with difficult people, you do not fall into the trap of ignoring the very basics of therapeutic communication. We often have the skills to deal with difficult situations but not the time to develop them. A good example of this is the common misconception by nurses that, in order to be able to care for aggressive patients, one needs to acquire specialist training in self-defence and 'restraint' only. While these issues may have their place as part of a much wider package of care in certain settings, nurses are commonly missing the point. The point being that basic communication skills such as accurate listening can be the most effective.

The 'rules' of communication are based, on the whole, on basic common sense, yet the simplest of skills are often sadly overlooked. One framework that best facilitates the development of such basic skills is that of Gerard Egan (1998). Egan's model, which offers three overall stages each with three identified steps, is a framework that lends itself naturally to nurse-related settings. This is particularly true as it covers exploration, understanding and action, and can be easily allied to the stages of the nursing process which include assessment, planning, implementation and evaluation. Although on initial examination Egan's (1998) 'The Skilled Helper' appears heavily theoretical, at times jargonated and somewhat complex in parts, the basic message is elementary. Before looking at the relevance of this helping model to nursing and therapeutic communication within health-related settings, let us first examine the model itself in more detail and its underlying principles.

Egan's model of helping

Gerard Egan's approach devised in the early 1980s is described as a problem management model. Although originally geared towards the world of counselling, Egan (1998) argues it is applicable to any context in which people need help. It is, therefore, not limited to the psychotherapeutic arena only but can easily be translated to the health care setting (Duxbury and Brown 1997). 'The approach is essentially a very general framework for helping, or more accurately for helping people to help themselves' (Davis and Fallowfield, 1994). The terms 'helping relationships' and 'helping models', although not new concepts, are fairly new expressions in the world of psychological approaches. Terminology can often be a minefield for any practitioner and, in the realms of psychology and related interventions, this is particularly apparent. One common complaint by nurses when exploring psychological approaches and communication skills, in general, is that health care professionals are not counsellors. This very much depends upon your interpretation of counselling. Classically our view of 'true counselling' is the concept of a trained therapist working with a client on a one-to-one basis at regular intervals and in a private and confidential setting. However, Nelson-Jones (1994) challenges this view and talks of both 'counselling relationships' whereby counselling is indeed the primary activity and 'helping relationships' in which 'counselling skills' are utilized but are only one part of the helper's relationship with the other person. The nurse–patient relationship clearly falls into the latter, particularly as basic counselling skills are crucial to this relationship. They include the ability to portray active listening, empathy, respect, genuineness and a non-judgemental approach, along with a variety of more advanced helping skills that will be addressed in more detail when exploring the work of Heron (1990).

Davis and Fallowfield (1994) argue that the term counselling can be directly applied to health care: 'Although counselling can be a direct source of help in enabling people to explore and understand their world more fully and therefore adapt more effectively, it is also a vehicle for making choices about other sources of direct help and treatment options'. Nelson-Jones (1983) has classified counselling into five types as follows:

- Developmental
- Problem focused
- Decision-making
- Crisis
- Supportive counselling.

None of these, he states, are mutually exclusive. The categories obviously relate to the intent of the counselling, differences in the type or types of problems and individuals involved. All categories are covered and encompassed in one form or another in the combined works of both Egan and Heron and hence their selection as a suggested approach in this practical text.

The focus of Egan's work is indeed upon helping and he is careful not to exclude practitioners or individuals by focusing upon the term counselling. A crucial assumption of Egan's work is that it is clearly recognized that people are responsible for their own behaviour and to some extent their situation. The implication of this is that you cannot solve people's problems for them but only help them to do so. This is particularly important when planning care and communicating with individuals deemed to be 'difficult'. The relationship between the helper and the individual is one of participation as opposed to direction. However, it is expected that the helper must take responsibility for and have a good working knowledge of the helping process. This is vital for the practitioner who is expected to adopt a variety of roles including listening, teaching, challenging, supporting, prescribing and advising (Davis and Fallowfield, 1994). It is imperative that the nurse has both the skills and the understanding to know when each role is appropriate and at what stage to intervene.

Egan (1998) emphasizes the need for clarity in the relationship from beginning to end. For this purpose he describes the process of helping as having three stages, each of which has specific requirements and gives specific direction. The model is hierarchical in that each stage builds upon what has been established at the previous level.

Stage one – problem clarification

The basic assumption of this stage is the recognition that in order to address problems effectively one must first have a full picture of the individual's experience and needs. Above all this requires 'exploration'. Exploration not only of how you as a nurse perceive the situation, but full exploration of the presenting problem(s) from the individual's own viewpoint. Egan, in fact, argues that the helper's understanding is not crucial to this stage, but becomes more important in stage 2. The individual with the problem is the main focus and Egan commonly refers to the importance of encouraging the person to 'tell their story'. We all have a story to tell and given the opportunity we like to be listened to. Allowing the individual to outline feelings, which are often not straightforward, takes time and an ability on the part of the helper to establish a trusting and supportive atmosphere (Davis and Fallowfield, 1994).

How the practitioner manages this early stage and steps involved will lay the crucial foundations for future progress and relations. It may well be the difference between a productive and healthy working partnership and the establishment of a difficult patient. As practitioners we have to take some responsibility for the therapeutic relationships we sometimes inadvertently make or break. Davis and Fallowfield (1994) argue 'this implies, the relationship between the person and helper is of central importance, and the aims of this and all subsequent stages are only likely to be achieved to the extent that a good working relationship is initially built and subsequently strengthened'.

In order to achieve the establishment of a fruitful therapeutic relationship, Egan (1998) suggests the utilization of certain fundamental qualities. Although important throughout all three stages of this model, these qualities are vital for the process of exploration and in helping the individual to recognize his or her problem areas. They include attentive and active listening skills, the use of reflection in the process of portraying empathy, probing to explore certain areas more fully and the ability to respond appropriately ensuring that both your verbal and non-verbal communications portray the same consistent message. It is crucial that the individual feels valued by the helper and one must be able to adopt a style that adequately gives a message of respect, genuineness and trust. Feeling these things and being able to communicate them are two separate things, the latter being the one that requires the most skill. The ability to portray to patients that you are interested in them, accepting of their needs and willing to help is reflected in the effective combination of good and accurate verbal and non-verbal communication skills. These are crucial foundations and building blocks for any nurse wishing to foster a therapeutic relationship and will be dealt with more fully later in this chapter. Once having mastered the basics and explored the patient's perception of his or her problem areas, the nurse is ready to facilitate the transition to stage two of Egan's model.

Stage two – setting goals

The aim of this stage relies heavily upon the work done in the previous stage; achieving a clearer overview of problem areas in order to be able to set some achievable goals. The reason the picture needs to be clearer is based on the premise that we do not always recognize our own problem areas, the part we have played in creating them or can play in the future in working through them. Sometimes our view of what has happened or is happening to us is distorted. Often we have a very narrow or one-sided picture of the situation. Whatever our predicament, the task of the helper is to enable individuals to develop a more useful and realistic understanding of the situation involving greater accuracy and objectivity (Davis and Fallowfield, 1994). This can be achieved because as practitioners, we are able to stand outside the situation, which may for the sufferer be loaded with pain, anxiety and disappointment.

In this capacity helpers can also identify possible blind spots, potential weaknesses and unused resources, giving a much fuller picture of the individual's situation other than the subjectivity of their own. Experience of the helping process and interventions that may be explored also provide a different view (or scenario as Egan calls them) of problems experienced. No man is an island and problems cannot be solved in isolation. Often it is the interrelation of a variety of factors that expose our vulnerability and health-related problems and the resulting need for help.

Once a better understanding of the scenario has been achieved based on information from the patient, significant others, and in light of observations and feedback from the nurse, the next step can be tackled. This involves helping the person to decide what he or she would like to achieve by way of managing the problems identified. This may involve setting a single goal or a series of sub-goals leading to a final desired outcome for more complex problems. Whatever the approach in relation to setting such goals, the goals formulated must be clear, specific, measurable, realistic, achievable and owned by the individual themselves (McFarlane and Castledine, 1982; Egan, 1998; Davis and Fallowfield, 1994). If goals are not set in this way, then often the patient will have difficulty moving on to the third stage of Egan's model, which involves facilitating action.

Stage three – facilitating action

The aim of this final stage is to put into operation ways of achieving goals previously set in stage two. This is a crucial stage and requires the nurse to be a catalyst rather than an activist. In many respects this is where nurses historically have tended to fall into difficulties. For many decades nurses have been socialized into doing everything for patients. It is only in recent years that it has been increasingly recognized that there are inherent dangers in such an approach, such as passivity and over-dependency (Walsh and Ford, 1992). By doing everything for patients there has been a limited need to give information, explain, promote health or educate and, as a result, patients have struggled once discharged from hospital. Today we are only too aware of the need to promote self-caring philosophies and behaviours (Orem, 1980) yet facilitation skills are still grossly underdeveloped and underused. This was highlighted in a study by Burnard and Morrison (1991) who found the majority of nurses relied most heavily upon prescriptive, informative and support-based skills (see Spotlight on Research No. 2). Other than support, Heron (1990) refers to these as authoritative skills and reflects the continued struggle we have in the health care system today with imbalances in power.

Spotlight on Research No. 2

Exploration of nurses' perceptions of their utilization of John Heron's Six Categories in practice (Burnard and Morrison, 1991)

This study aimed to find out whether or not there was a consistency in the way nurses viewed their interpersonal skills in terms of Heron's analysis.

Methodology

Subjects A convenience sample was used of 117 trained nurses who attended counselling skills workshops run by one of the authors of this study. These nurses were from the fields of general, psychiatric and community nursing.

Design This was essentially a quantitative survey using objective data.

Method Following a period of introduction and familiarization with the category analysis, the nurses were invited to take part in the study by completing a rating scale that ranged from scores of 1 to 5. Nurses were asked to rate how they perceived their skills in each of Heron's six categories.

1 = Not skilled
5 = Very skilled.

Analysis Once the rating scales had been completed, a matrix was used consisting of rows and columns. Each row represented a respondent and each column represented a category of analysis. From this matrix, calculations of mean rating scores for each of the categories were possible and from these the six categories practitioners ranked themselves as 'least skilled–most skilled'.

Findings

Findings were as follows: The category that respondents felt most skilled in using was the supportive category (mean rating score 4.23, rank order 1). The information category was in second position (mean rating score 3.94, rank order 2). Third was the prescriptive category (mean rating score 3.75, rank order 3). The catalytic category was ranked next (mean rating score 3.3, rank order 4) followed by the cathartic category (mean rating score 2.37, rank order 5). The confronting category was in last position.

continued

continued
This rank order mirrors exactly previous studies exploring the same (Burnard and Morrison, 1989).

Discussion

This study supports the suggestion that nurses are generally more skilled in being supportive, informative and prescriptive and less skilled in being catalytic, cathartic and confronting.

Suggestions for these trends include the following:

1. The organizational culture in hospitals may work against the development of a facilitative style.
2. The facilitative approach takes too much time.
3. Catalytic, cathartic and confronting approaches involve investment of self, which may be emotionally draining.
4. Nursing often involves practical activities that involve 'getting the work done' (Melia, 1987).
5. There has been a considerable emphasis upon the information giving aspect of nursing, which may account for some of the emphasis on this category.

Conclusion

It is notable that contrary to Heron's authoritative/facilitative dichotomy, the nurses in this study aligned the confronting interventions with cathartic and catalytic ones, thus deviating from Heron's original formula. This may offer an insight into training needs and the difficulty nurses have in meeting patients' emotional needs. It is significant that nurses perceive themselves as being most skilled in being supportive which is the skill that appears to underpin all others. This may be a starting point for future interpersonal skills training.

Based on
Burnard, P. and Morrison, P. (1991) *Caring and Communicating*. London: Macmillan.

Davis and Fallowfield (1994) argue the key to an action stage is to have a good knowledge of and review the various ways of reaching specific goals. Expertise is important and to be able to make careful selection of chosen approach(es), to be prepared for any difficulties that may emerge, to prepare the patient appropriately and then to provide support and ongoing encouragement while they are being carried out. Facilitation is an art and it is not about opting out or letting the patient get on with it. It requires knowledge and skill and is time consuming, requiring preparation and supervision time. Evaluation is then crucial and is not necessarily an end point in itself, but more often the beginning, as a new cycle may begin following feedback.

Egan argues there are two specific groups of skills involved in this very skilful stage. These are:

- Programme development skills which involve the brainstorming of possible avenues to problem solving and resulting action.
- Facilitation action skills which involve helping the person to make the preparations necessary to carry out the plans. This includes anticipation of potential difficulties and assisting the individual to acquire both the necessary skills and information.

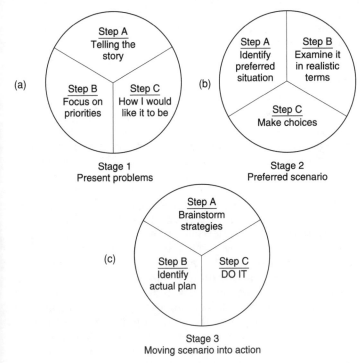

Fig 2.1a–c Overview of the three Stages and Sub Steps (adapted from Egan 1998)

Fundamental skills of therapeutic communication

Communication is undoubtedly a two-way process. 'An intervention where two or more people both send and receive massages and in the process both present themselves and interpret the other' (Peel, 1995). One cannot fail to communicate and messages are continuously sent both verbally and non-verbally, intentionally and otherwise. Although we do not speak all the time and are selective in when we choose to verbalize and when we do not, non-verbal behaviour is ongoing and not always so easily or selectively displayed. Non-verbal communication is at times evident without recognition or intent and, although we largely aim to complement what we say with what we do, this is not always the case. Argyle (1990) has argued that non-verbal communication has five times as much effect on a person's understanding of a message compared with words. As such it is important that we recognize what we are communicating and the possible avenues by which we communicate. Davis (1994) highlights this point and suggests that 'non verbal communication affects the behaviour between nurse and patient and so influences the care given'. The five avenues of non-verbal communication are:

- Facial movements
- Eye contact
- Body posture and movement
- Touch
- Personal space.

We generally assume that behaviour involving one or all of the above factors has some meaning attached to it. These assumptions are, in turn, based on a host of factors. For instance, how well we know the individual who is communicating; what our relationship is with them; the situational and cultural context at any given moment in time; gender; past experience; and our ability to interpret information, e.g. sight, hearing, knowledge, perception. Once we have made assumptions about the behaviour, we then react accordingly. Of course verbal content will always be a big influencing factor when making those assumptions, if speech is an accompanying factor. Let me give you an example. If somebody were to sneak up behind you and suddenly put their hand over your eyes without saying anything, you would have every reason to be scared, particularly if you were in an unfamiliar place. On the other hand, if a friend were to do the same to you and say 'surprise' and you recognized the voice, your reaction would, more than likely, be different.

Many nurses, it would seem, struggle to take the problem of effective communication seriously. Health care professionals appear to be of the view that communication is both straightforward and easy (Davis, 1994). Yet time and time again clinicians are criticized for their poor and inadequate communication skills (Ley, 1989; Hadfield-Law, 1998). Patients are increasingly dissatisfied (Rogers *et al.*, 1993). Once nurses are ready to examine self and acknowledge that therapeutic communication at its best is a skilled activity that can be developed and warrants ongoing practice and evaluation, then the learning process can begin to the benefit of nurse–patient communication. In order to graduate successfully to more advanced levels in any given helping model, the building blocks of therapeutic communication must be openly practised and reaffirmed. These are the basic skills of therapeutic communication, the most fundamental of which involves the ability to 'attend' to patients fully and 'actively' listen. Patients rate the need to be listened to very high on the agenda of helping behaviours and this elementary skill involves the effective and complementary use of both verbal and non-verbal behaviours. These behaviours are commonly termed 'attending skills'.

Attending skills

Attending skills involve the ability to use non-verbal signals that communicate the giving of attention by means of eye contact, head nods, facial expression and appropriate cues. Arnold and Boggs (1995) refer to this process as 'presence'. They suggest that 'presence' or 'attending' is the ability of the nurse to remain physically, spiritually and emotionally attuned to a client's communication and being. Attending behaviours, therefore, invite the client to communicate with the nurse and demonstrate interest and, above all, a sincere desire to understand. Gardener (1992) described it as a 'gift of self' which reflects the total attention and time one focuses upon another. To be 'attended to' is a warming experience and one that can instil a feeling of self-worth in the receiver.

Active listening

This includes the process of 'attending', but takes the concept of hearing and communicating what you hear to a much deeper level. It is a dynamic process, whereby one person hears a message, decides upon its meaning and conveys an understanding about the meaning to the sender (Arnold and Boggs, 1995).

Listening is not always straightforward or uncomplicated. It is an active process concerned with receiving largely aural stimuli (DeVito, 1986). In order to fully understand the concept of active listening, one must first be able to appreciate that listening can also be a very passive process.

Passive listening

Passive listening requires far less time and energy and largely involves 'lying back and letting something happen' (Dainow and Bailey, 1992). It is highlighted by 'non-attending' and is often without response or with inaccurate response (Stewart, 1993). As with active listening, passive listening can be portrayed both verbally and non-verbally. For instance, think back to times when you have been at a lecture and not actively listening to the speaker. What were you thinking, feeling, doing? It may be that you were daydreaming about something else, were slumped down in your chair, and looking out of the window or that you remained silent and uninvolved. You were not attending. Then, suddenly, the lecturer calls your name and asks you a question. Your posture immediately changes to that of an attentive one and you have to become mentally and physically responsive in preparation for active listening. Can you see the difference?

DeVito (1986) argues passive listening is not always without its merits and some recognition is warranted. For instance, listening without talking and directing can be a powerful way of communicating acceptance or that you feel at ease with someone. It also allows the speaker to develop his or her own thoughts and feelings without judgement or intrusion, using you as a 'sounding board', so to speak. Finally, passive listening can be very relaxing both mentally and physically and may involve just listening to music.

Because we listen to different people for different reasons, the principles we follow in listening effectively should naturally vary from situation to situation. However, the art of effective listening in interpersonal situations is to be an active participant. This includes expressing both verbally and non-verbally that we are listening through what we endeavour to say and what we do. Therefore, active listening incorporates the process of 'attending' in a largely behavioural sense but requires greater mental and physical preparation and participation (DeVito, 1986).

Active listening

Dainow and Bailey (1992) argue that active listening is 'disciplined listening' as opposed to 'in one ear and out the other'. They also highlight the fact that we have two ears and only one mouth, therefore, listening and speaking should be on a ratio of 2:1.

For most people listening is a natural activity. However, distinguishing between our 'inner voice' and 'interference' (things we think about when listening), and 'outer listening' is something we must learn and very much a part of our socialization. It is important that nurses learn to listen effectively if they are to understand what is being transmitted by patients. Only then can an accurate, supportive response be given. This involves thinking critically and choosing responses that will facilitate greater understanding of the client's perspective (Egan, 1986). It includes the integration of a host of factors such as the following:

- Non-verbal cues
- Tone of voice
- Intuition
- Previous conversations (Arnold and Boggs, 1995).

It is also important that the nurse not only listens actively but is able to portray this to the patient. Egan (1998) advocates the use of 'SOLER' to facilitate this. This approach is a key feature of the stage one exploration phase in his helping model. Although a very basic recipe, it incorporates and captivates the crucial elements of 'attending' effectively.

S – Sit 'squarely' to your patient
O – Adopt an 'open' posture
L – 'Lean' slightly forward
E – Maintain good 'eye contact'
R – Endeavour to portray a 'relaxed' approach.

Many might choose to miss the point of such a simple outline. The most productive way to utilize approaches such as these is to integrate the basic format into your own approach and way of doing things. The main aim is to show concern and interest in an accepting and relaxed atmosphere. It is not about putting yourself into positions that feel unreal and unnatural to you, but about recognizing the importance of what you say and what you do in establishing a bond and trusting relationship. SOLER largely emphasizes the non-verbal elements of active listening, yet when you are listening, the intermittent verbal messages you give back to the patient must be recognized also and valued for their importance. Nelson-Jones (1994) focuses more fully on the verbal elements of effective communication.

Verbal messages

In order to listen actively, your verbal as well as non-verbal communication is important. In fact, on the whole, it is rare to detach one from the other. Along with voice type and tone, the content of what is being said is crucial. One of the most common faults displayed by practitioners is the act of speaking too quickly and too softly (Heron, 1990). This often indicates anxiety which, in turn, may make the patient feel anxious (Nelson-Jones, 1994). Conversely, when listening to a client, verbal speed and quietness may alert the nurse to the patient's increasing levels of anxiety.

A useful tool when developing your own personal style of listening and verbal encouragement and to assist you when determining what to listen out for, is the following acronym devised by Nelson-Jones (1994) – VAPER:

V – Volume
A – Articulation
P – Pitch
H – Emphasis
R – Rate.

Volume gives much away in terms of level of emotion and arousal. When one is angry, volume naturally increases and certain words may be emphasized more than others indicating areas to focus upon.

Rate and pitch also commonly increase when anxious or upset. Articulation or the ability to make oneself understood can be affected. Difficulty expressing oneself can be an indication of distress, particularly when discussing emotive areas. VAPER can give away many clues to the active listener and can be a useful framework on which to role model a calm, informative, clear and relaxed way of communicating. A calm and warm voice can be most reassuring and promote an atmosphere of trust and sharing. As such, VAPER can assist the nurse in his or her therapeutic communication and facilitate expression from patients.

Additional verbal skills can also assist the active listening process and prompt patients to share their thoughts more openly. A combination of skills is recommended and includes the use of openers, small rewards and open-ended questions (Nelson-Jones, 1994). Each require the use of a few words only and accurate voice and body messages.

Openers

These are relatively straightforward and are used either to open a conversation or in response to a patient's behaviour or situation. The message contained in all of them is 'I am interested and prepared to listen'.

Examples
'You seem a bit down today, is there something on your mind?'
'Would you like to talk about it?'
'How are you, how was your day?'
'Hello I'm.................. Tell me a little about why you're here?'

Your tone of voice and body message must be congruent with your verbal messages in order to be effective. Often you will find you have your own natural openers that you commonly use. However, with some thought, you might find something more effective. Some patients may find it difficult to talk straight away and may feel nervous and unsure. Therefore, the use of silence and 'follow up' remarks can be beneficial. For example:

'Take your time'
'I know it's pretty hard to get started'.

Setting the scene in any relationship is all-important and first impressions really do count. Encouraging a patient to open up on that initial meeting, when vulnerable or at any point in your relationship is crucial and a most valuable building block. Openers, although extremely simplistic, warrant some careful thought and reflection, particularly when evaluating your own skills. Do you tend to have a problem starting people off and if you do, could you take the lead and open discussions more effectively?

Once having mastered the art of using effective openers and follow-up prompts, the use of 'small rewards' can be an additional verbal communication tool.

Small rewards

These are brief verbal expressions of interest from the listener designed to encourage the speaker. They convey the message 'Please go on, I am with you'.

Examples include:
Um – hmn
Please continue
Tell me more
Go on
I see

Oh
And...
Really...
Sure...
So...
Ah
Yes

Another form of small reward is to repeat the last word or few words spoken back to someone in the form of a question. So, for instance, if a patient said to you. 'I feel so angry with him for what he did', you might want to repeat the phrase in the form of a question 'What he did?'. This shows you are listening attentively and interested and encourages the individual to expand upon something that is obviously painful.

Thirdly, open questions are a very useful prompt and valuable throughout any stage of a helping relationship.

Open questions

These may be used to encourage individuals to elaborate upon their internal viewpoints or to get them to expand into an area you feel is important based on your active listening. If you have been listening accurately you will build up a picture of problem areas that are commonly referred to or avoided altogether. Either way they may warrant further exploration (Nelson-Jones, 1994).

Open-ended questions are open to interpretation and cannot be answered by yes, no or a one-worded response. They usually begin with 'How, what, where, when, in what way or can you tell me?' A variation of the open-ended question is the focused question, which limits the response to certain areas but again requires more than just a yes/no answer. This approach is particularly useful when specific information is needed rather than broad and vague responses that may not be immediately relevant.

For instance, 'can you tell me more about the pain in your arm?'.

Focused questions may be particularly useful if time is limited or specific information needed. However, they should not take the place of open questions when warranted. Whatever the context, two people in conversation are normally exercising their own egos. We all like to talk about ourselves while listening to others with only half an ear (Nelson-Jones, 1994). In effective communication the focus of the listener remains fully on the speaker. At appropriate moments the listener actively checks with the speaker the accuracy of their understanding of what they have heard (Hobbs, 1992).

This leads on to a second major basic skill called empathy that can be developed considerably with experience and practice. There are two forms of empathy. There is a basic kind and an advanced empathy.

Basic empathy

Empathy in its most fundamental sense involves understanding the experience, behaviours and feelings of others as they experience them. It means helpers must try to put aside their own biases, prejudices and points of view and enter the world of the client in order to develop a feeling for their inner world (Egan, 1998). It is, simplistically, putting yourself into somebody else's shoes. Rogers (1980) defines it as 'entering the private, perceptual world of another and becoming thoroughly at home in it'. It involves being sensitive, moment by moment, to the changing felt meanings.

Helpers, in the intensity of their listening and being with their clients, sometimes see more clearly what clients only half see or hint at. This deeper kind of empathy involves 'sensing meanings of which the client is scarcely aware' (Rogers, 1980).

Example
For instance, a client talks about his anger at his wife, but as he talks, the helper hears not just anger but also the hurt. It may be that someone can talk with relative ease about their anger but not about feelings of hurt. Empathetic listeners ask themselves such questions as 'what is this person only half saying'.

It is all about intuition. However, empathy is not just the ability to enter into and understand the world of another person but also to be able to communicate this understanding to him or her (Egan, 1998). It is a skill that is highly valued by Egan and one that spans the boundaries of both stage one and stage two of his model.

Egan (1998) argues that empathy involves:

- 'Being' with others
- Showing professional presence
- Development of a basic communication skill that can be learnt.

Gladstein (1983) suggests there are two kinds of basic empathy:

Emotional empathy – This is the ability to be affected emotionally by another person's state, for example to become sad when we hear of someone else's misfortunes.

Role taking empathy – The ability to understand another person's state, condition, frame of reference or point of view. 'Role taking empathy', suggests Gladstein (1983), is the most crucial in initiating the helping process, establishing rapport and developing closeness. This helps clients to identify problems and to explore themselves and their situations. While this form of empathy can be learnt (Egan, 1998), emotional empathy is something you may or may not feel depending upon the individual, the experience and the moment in time. However, it is no good feeling and understanding another's experience if you cannot communicate your feeling of empathy to them.

Nelson-Jones (1993) prefers not to use the word empathy but instead talks of *reflective responding* which he defines as 'responding with understanding as if in the client's internal viewpoint'. He suggests this not only involves feeling for and understanding your client but also 'mirroring with your verbal voice and body messages what you see and hear'.

The term is preferred for two main reasons:

1. The term reflection more closely describes the process involved rather than empathy, whereby you reflect words back to the patient in order to clarify your level of understanding.
2. The term avoids confusion with Rogers' use of empathy who believes it to be an attitude only rather than a skill.

Egan (1998) argues it is both an attitude and a skill and this debate continues. However, helping models largely support the latter view that empathy is a skill that can be developed and applied to various settings.

Helping skills necessary for empathy

The main skills involved in the portrayal of empathy are:
- Reflection
- Rewording
- Reflective feelings
- Reflecting feelings and reasons
- Clarification
- Probing.

Reflection and clarification
Skilled helpers are very sharp at picking up clients' feelings.

Reflecting feelings is built upon the ability to *reword* – both reflecting feelings and rewording involve what the patient has said or indicated to you and rephrasing the gist of the meaning back to them but in your own words. It is not about just repeating phrases. Rewording alone has distinct limitations. The nurse or helper must look beyond superficial words to find feelings and reasons also.

Example
Clients may send voice and body messages that qualify or negate verbal messages. Paul says 'I'm okay', yet speaks softly and has tears in his eyes. A good reflection of feelings picks up these messages and reflects them back to the client. If the nurse were just to accept what Paul was saying at face value, crucial issues would be missed with a general lack of understanding (Nelson-Jones, 1993).

Basic rewording
Examples
Parent: 'I told my kids to go to hell.'
Nurse: 'You were really angry with them.'

Employee: 'Some of the time I like working here, but some of the time I'm less positive.'
Manager: 'You have mixed feelings about what you do here.'

A good rewording of verbal content can provide mirror reflections that are clearer than the original statements. Clients may show appreciation and feel that you are in tune with them, 'That's right', 'you've got me'.

A simple tip for rewording is to start your responses with: 'You...'

Reflecting feelings
Rewording is a basic technique used mainly to reflect verbal content. However, the language of feelings is not just words. Reflecting feelings is being in tune with a client's flow of emotions and experience and being able to communicate this back to them. Inadequately distinguishing between thoughts and feelings can be a problem for both clients and helpers. The distinction is important both in reflecting feelings and also when helping clients to influence how they feel by altering how they think. Constant reflective responding focusing on feelings runs the risk of encouraging clients to wallow in feelings rather than to move on to how best to deal with them (Nelson-Jones, 1993). Reflecting feelings

involves both receiver and sender skills (Egan, 1998). In other words what the nurse observes and understands and what he or she says and does in response.

Picking up incongruent voice and body messages
Information about clients' feelings does not necessarily come from what they say but from how they say it. Sometimes the verbal, voice and body messages clients send are congruent; however, more often than not, clients' messages are heavily encoded (hidden). Clients may struggle to express what they truly feel because of their conditioning about what they should feel. It takes time to be able to trust helpers. Effective helpers have a 'third ear' to detect what is left unsaid or camouflaged (core messages) (Egan, 1998). Patience rather than pressure is important and comments and prompts such as:

'I think I hear what you're saying...'
'...Am I right?' (clarification).
'I'm not altogether clear what you're saying to me.'

Or

'I'm getting mixed messages from you. On the one hand you are saying you don't mind, while on the other hand you seem tearful. Are you putting on a brave face?'
 This is the core skill of clarification and is an ongoing and integral part of reflection.
 When reflecting feelings there are two key stages:

1. First you have to decode the overall message accurately using any of the above techniques.
2. Secondly you must formulate an emotionally expressive reflective response that communicates back the crux of the client's feelings.

To do that you must endeavour to:

• Send back the crux of the clients' message
• Be sensitive to client's underlying feelings and agendas
• Keep your response simple
• Use voice and body messages to add expressiveness to your verbal message(s)
• State client's main feeling at the start of your response (You feel...)
• Check your understanding (Am I right?) (Nelson-Jones, 1993).

Reflecting feelings and reasons

A useful variation of reflective responding, says Nelson-Jones (1993), is to reflect both feelings and the reasons for them. This does not mean that you make your own interpretation or offer an explanation from your external viewpoint but, instead, use the client's reasons for a feeling.

Here the helper's 'You feel...because' response shows greater understanding and listening, helps clients tell their stories and reveals how clients' thinking contributes to unwanted feelings.

Egan (1998) suggests the following tips for improving the quality of empathy:

1. Give yourself time to think – don't jump in!
2. Use short responses – it is the client you want to engage in dialogue.
3. Gear your responses to the individual client and share their emotional tone. For instance, if she is angry or sad, share that you have noticed this with her.

He further identifies some common problems that practitioners encounter when developing empathy skills:

1. Using poor substitutes for empathy such as no response, a question whereby you ignore the feeling, a cliché, an interpretation or moving straight into action when this is really part of the exploration stage.
2. Counterfeits of accurate empathy such as inaccurate empathy, pretending to understand, or parroting, which means just repeating back word for word what somebody says to you. This serves no real purpose.

In most of the examples used so far in the discussion of empathy, clients have demonstrated a willingness to explore themselves freely. While it is essential that helpers respond empathetically for those who do not reveal feelings, it is also necessary at times to encourage and prompt those individuals. Therefore, the ability to use prompts and probes (verbal tactics for helping clients talk about themselves and define their problems more specifically) is another important skill.

Using probes

This involves:

- Using open questions that help a client talk more freely or clarifying statements as discussed earlier.
- The 'accent' which involves a one or two word restatement that highlights part of the previous client response.

- Minimal prompts (uh-huh, head nods, yes, etc.) called small rewards.

Some cautions in the use of probes
- Do not overuse them.
- Once you have used a probe or prompt, give time to let the client respond.

After using a probe, use basic empathy rather than a series of probes. After all, if a probe is effective, it will yield relevant information that then needs to be listened to and understood (Egan, 1998).

When students and practitioners are first introduced to the skills highlighted, many express reservations such as:

'It's so unnatural!'
'Clients will just think I'm repeating everything they say!'
'It gets in the way of being spontaneous!'
'It makes me feel too self-conscious' (Nelson-Jones, 1993).

The key to using the skills identified so far, is to integrate the basics into your own repertoire, language, and way of doing things. In this way it will be more real to you and more believable to the patient. Reflective responding and related skills should not be something you use all the time, they should instead be flexibly incorporated into your helping skills repertoire. However, they are particularly useful on the following occasions:

- When creating a safe emotional climate for clients to tell their stories
- When you need to show that you have understood
- When you need to check that you have understood
- When clients appear to be struggling to get in touch with their thoughts and feelings
- When clients need a reward or emotional stepping stone to continue talking
- When you need to check clients' understanding of specific points you make (Nelson-Jones 1993).

Overall, many helpers use the terms empathy and reflection or rephrasing interchangeably. Egan (1998) argues that empathy is much more than a communication skill, but a 'way of being'. It requires a strong need to understand your patient and is not just simply a behavioural response when used in its truest form. Once having mastered the art of communicating empathy, advanced empathy may be developed. For some, this comes very naturally and is partly based on intuition.

Advanced empathy

This is a term highlighted by Egan (1998) and involves giving expression to that which the client only implies. This involves finding feelings and meanings that are buried, hidden or beyond the immediate reach of the client. It is an ongoing process that involves 'piecing together' relevant information and experiences from the helping relationship. Advanced empathy can be communicated in a number of different ways as follows:

1. Expressing what is only implied once rapport has been established.
2. Identifying themes, patterns of behaviour and/or emotion. For instance, you may notice that a patient seems to be experiencing:
   (a) poor self-image
   (b) dominance and the need for power
   (c) helplessness.
3. Connecting islands – this means helping clients to make connections or fill the gaps between emotions and behaviours. It may be that you notice they become angry or upset at certain times or when discussing certain people or situations.
4. From the less to the more – in this instance unclear issues are clarified and built upon. Greater understanding is achieved between nurse and patient as you explore issues with them and ask for clarification or check out uncertainties. Don't be afraid to get the clearest possible picture you can. If you don't understand, say so. By role modelling such behaviour, the client too may feel more able to ask questions and clarify when unsure.

In summary, skills such as those addressed are commonly employed at a very early stage in the development of the nurse–patient relationship or helping work. Hobbs (1992) identifies them as basic skills.

Basic skills are fundamental to effective communication and include:

1. Attending behaviour
2. Use of open and closed questions
3. Selective and active listening
4. Reflection of feelings.

The skill of empathy, Hobbs (1992) proposes, is more easily developed at an intermediate stage of the relationship when it is anticipated that a bond will have been created between nurse and patient.

Egan's framework is more structured and identifies a systematic format for problem solving that includes the three stages of exploration, understanding and goal setting in action. Egan (1998) suggests that certain skills are needed for each stage but argues that there is adequate scope for flexibility, individual preference and creativity in the chosen treatment approach. For instance, information-giving skills in stage two can be translated into a variety of approaches. One patient may prefer a nurse to demonstrate a skill while another may wish to have the opportunity to speak to other patients who are successfully managing similar problems. Egan's model of helping, therefore, offers both structure and adaptability when developing your therapeutic communication skills and knowledge.

To complement Egan's approach, John Heron's six-category intervention analysis framework (SCIA) provides the ideal companion. Heron (1990) provides the practitioner with an array of valuable tools that can be applied throughout each stage and step of Egan's model. Therefore this combination provides the framework, foundation and manual of tools necessary to be an effective communicator. Such a marriage can be integrated into your day-to-day practice and can be used specifically for those patients who present with either difficult behaviour or problems.

Before exploring suggested strategies for working with difficult patients in the following chapter, an overview of Heron's framework is presented and the intervention categories outlined.

Heron's Six Category Intervention Analysis Framework (SCIA)

John Heron first established this framework for counselling interventions in the mid-1970s. Although originally developed to explore the management styles of institutions (Blake and Morton, 1972), Heron revised and enlarged upon this model to incorporate a range of tools. However, he now argues that its comprehensive repertoire of interventions facilitate its application to a broad range of occupational groups (Heron, 1990; Brown and Duxbury, 1997). It has since been widely used in an array of settings and has become an important ingredient in, or the basis of, interpersonal skills training for many health care professions. Heron (1990) argues the framework can be used by any 'practitioner' who is offering a professional service to a client. A client being any person who is freely choosing (in most cases) to avail him- or herself of the practitioner's service in order to meet some particular need. Between practitioner and client there is a mutually agreed voluntary contract implicit in the relationship. However, this may not always be formal or visible. The nurse–patient relationship is a good example of the practitioner–client partnership.

Inherent within this relationship there may be fluctuating dynamics. As a result, the contract agreed between practitioner and client may become confused, ill-defined or unfamiliar. This can lead to stress and may even precipitate an increase in the numbers of difficult patients or at least difficult encounters. Before Heron's framework can be used to its potential, the central issue of the enabling relationship, and how it will operate, must be identified, clarified and mutually agreed. Then and only then, can nurse and patient begin to communicate effectively and work towards therapeutic goals. This is the basis for therapeutic communication.

The six categories adapted by John Heron are identified to help the practitioner to meet the individual needs of patients or respond to their behaviours. Helpers select one of six categories of intervention most suited to the individual and their situation within which there is a choice of roles. For instance, if a patient is lacking in information there is a range of information-giving skills to choose from, if someone needs additional support there are support-giving skills. If a patient is struggling to express him- or herself, there is a collection of tools to assist in this expression and so forth.

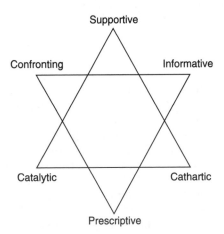

Figure 2.2 The six categories of counselling intervention (from Heron, 1990). Reprinted by permission of Sage Publications Ltd.

In researching human need and experience, Heron (1990) argues he has captured every possible client need and practitioner role under the broad umbrella of the six categories of intervention. In order to explore these categories more fully, an overview of each is now presented.

Authoritative categories

1. *Prescriptive interventions* – a prescriptive intervention seeks to direct the behaviour of the client and therefore it is often instructional in type. It involves giving direction or advice to the client about what he or she should do when the practitioner is not or will not be around.
2. *Informative interventions* – an informative intervention seeks to impart knowledge, information or meaning to the client. This may involve new material, revision, clarification of points already addressed or updating old information.
3. *Confrontational interventions* – a confronting intervention seeks to raise the client's consciousness about some limiting attitude or behaviour of which they may be relatively unaware. Of all the categories this appears to be one of the most difficult to utilize confidently (Burnard and Morrison, 1991). Yet if used skilfully, it can be one of the most beneficial, especially when caring for difficult patients. This category is not about being aggressive but about assisting the individual to recognize their weaknesses in light of their strengths. This must be done in an atmosphere of support with the necessary assistance and strategies to facilitate progress.

Facilitative categories

4. *Cathartic interventions* – a cathartic intervention seeks to enable the client to discharge, to abreact (release) painful emotion, be it grief, fear or anger. The health care setting is rich with both expressed and repressed emotions. Yet the expression of emotion is often stifled, restricted, avoided, ignored or blatantly disallowed (Menzies, 1968; Smith and Hart, 1994). Repressed stress and frustration is increasingly believed to be responsible for a whole range of health-related problems (Ogden, 1998), therefore, this is one area it is crucial that practitioners become more skilled in.

Health care professionals are often afraid to allow patients to unleash their emotions for fear that the individual will then become out of control. This is fear of the unknown. It may also be that we are afraid of our own emotion. In reality, even when expressing emotion, it is rare for an individual's distress to escalate out of control particularly if and when the supporting individual displays effective communication skills. Imagine those times when you have gone home and shut the door and for whatever reason sobbed uncontrollably. Do you continue to sob in the same vein indefinitely? No! More often than not we re-contain our emotion almost as quickly as we have unleashed it and often feel so much better for having done so! Fear of emotion is a state of mind and this is one category we must particularly strive to develop in the health care setting.

5. *Catalytic interventions* – a catalytic intervention seeks to elicit self-discovery, self-care, learning and problem solving in the client. The emphasis in health care has shifted now and patient participation is both expected and encouraged in practice (Brearley, 1990). Giving patients the skills to function independently is our ultimate aim.

6. *Supportive interventions* – a supportive intervention seeks to affirm the worth and value of a client, their qualities, attitudes and behaviour. This is one aspect, as carers, we tend naturally to excel in. It is also the one category that is vital to all the other categories and closely interrelates. Support is crucial to all avenues of nursing, all patients, whatever their need, situation or setting.

Spotlight on Research No. 3

An investigation into the meaning and nature of the term catharsis (McGregor Kettles, 1994)

Nurses are encouraged to use catharsis and cathartic techniques as part of their clinical practice to enable clients and themselves to release emotion, to feel better and to facilitate coping. However, the literature does not provide clinical nursing evidence for its use. Many writers argue that the concept of emotion should have a greater role in the behavioural sciences than they currently enjoy (Gordon, 1990; Heron, 1990).

Background

Nurses work with clients in therapeutic situations on a daily basis and emotional well-being is now a recognized part of care (George, 1991). Catharsis is used by some

continued

continued

nurses in the delivery of care, but what do nurses believe about catharsis? Are nurses perpetuating the myths about catharsis such as the unquestionable merits of 'getting emotions out' (Tarvis, 1982). The main purpose of this investigation is to examine the beliefs about and understanding of catharsis which two groups of nurses hold.

Methodology

Design A survey was used to discover what nurses believe about and understand by the term 'catharsis' and to investigate whether age, sex, philosophical viewpoint and nursing qualifications influence the answers given.

Subjects The sample included 142 nurse respondents (49 teachers and 93 students). A student population was drawn from various courses including post enrolled conversion, the 3-year RMN course and the Diploma in Nursing Studies (Common Foundation Programme and the Mental Health Branch).

Method A self-administration questionnaire was used. This included one qualitative question about understanding of the term catharsis and 16 statements regarding the beliefs nurses hold about catharsis. Statements included such areas as the beliefs about expression of emotions, about the role of cognitions in and about the role of therapeutic catharsis. On a five point Likert-type scale respondents indicated the extent to which they agreed or disagreed with the statements

Analysis Most of the information gathered was either nominal or ordinal, which meant that all statistical analyses had to be carried out using non-parametric techniques. Chi-square and the Kruskal-Wallis one way analysis of variance were the analytical tools of choice.

Findings

As many as 95% of students accepted that expressing emotion was beneficial, while some qualified nurses questioned its value (19%). Results showed that sex (male), qualifications and level of training have strong relationships with the view that catharsis is negative. Male student nurses hold more mixed or behaviourist philosophical views whereas female nurses at all ages tend to be more humanistic in their beliefs.

The main categories to emerge from respondents' responses to the question 'what do you understand by the word catharsis?' were: (a) release of emotion (n = 71), (b) expression of feelings (n = 38) and other (n = 33). The terms distress and discharge did not feature.

Conclusion

Two thirds of the nurses surveyed at all levels have some degree of understanding of what catharsis means. In addition, the psychotherapeutic value for clinical practice was largely clear; however, the social context in which catharsis occurs is not. A variety of demographics do influence views about catharsis as highlighted and despite nurses as a group claiming to believe in humanistic values, emotional catharsis as a central therapeutic goal is not endorsed without question.

Based on
McGregor Kettles, A. (1994) Catharsis: an investigation of its meaning and nature. *Journal of Advanced Nursing*, **20**, 368–376.

You may have noticed that the six categories fall within two much broader headings; authoritative and facilitative. Heron (1990) argues that 'the authoritative interventions are neither more nor less useful and valuable than the facilitative ones. It all depends on the nature of the practitioner's role, the particular needs of the client, and the content or focus of the intervention'. The first three are termed authoritative because the practitioner or nurse, in this case, largely takes a lead role in the care. This involves guiding, giving instruction and raising awareness. It ultimately requires the nurse to take the initiative and resulting responsibility when the patient is not able to do so for him- or herself. This may be due to a lack of knowledge, limited ability or poor motivation. Authoritative interventions may be more commonly used in the early stages of the nurse–patient relationship depending upon level of need or disability, transcending to more facilitative approaches later on. However, this would not be the case in confrontation, which is more effective if your relationship with a patient is established.

Facilitative interventions, by comparison, seek to enable clients to become more autonomous and take more responsibility for themselves. This may involve giving them the knowledge, information and skills to do this, by affirming their worth and value or by releasing the emotional pain that appears to be blocking their personal power (Heron, 1990).

No one category carries more weight than another nor do you need to use them in any order of sequence. You will naturally rely more heavily upon one or two as opposed to others by the nature of a patient's needs and responses. Each of these categories is valuable when intervening with patients generally, but they are the foundation, in conjunction with Egan's basic skills, for communicating more therapeutically with patients perceived to be 'difficult'.

When using Heron's model there are some general points that need to be recognized and understood.

- In the first instance, Heron (1990) argues this framework is not a rigid dogma to be added to without question or evaluation. He, in fact, advocates that it is essential to check, recheck, amend, select and modify as need be. Some of his recommended approaches are not suitable for day-to-day use within nurse-related settings and only those deemed to be practical have been identified in this book.
- Secondly, the categories can be applied with some confidence in that they have clearly stood the test of time and appear to be exhaustive in the intervention categories that can be used in a helping relationship.
- Thirdly, there is no real hierarchical value among the categories. Although there are significant areas of overlap between some categories, supportive interventions that might be catalytic or cathartic for example, the six categories are independent of each other.
- Fourthly, having identified that the categories themselves appear exhaustive, the suggested interventions within are not and allow for the skills, knowledge, ability and creativity of the individual practitioner.

- Finally, the focus of the relationship is one to one: that of helper and helped and the special relationship that ensues. This in itself raises issues for the nursing profession and chosen organization of care in any given setting. In order to develop an effective and therapeutic relationship there needs to be an investment of time, consistency, the establishment of trust and rapport and an ongoing understanding of the individual's needs.

A consistent approach is paramount when using Heron's framework. In addition, Heron (1990) advocates that the skilled practitioner ideally is someone who:

1. Is equally proficient in a wide range of interventions in each of the categories. A small team and good skill mix may be advantageous.
2. Can move elegantly, flexibly and clearly from one intervention to another as necessary.
3. Is aware at any given time of which intervention they are using and why.
4. Knows when to lead the client and when to follow.
5. Has and understands a balance between power over the client (advocacy), power shared with the client and the facilitation of client power.

Supervision, communication, training and support are crucial to the practitioner using this framework and working on a one-to-one basis with a patient. This is especially important for nurses working with patients who have many difficulties or who are proving to be 'difficult' themselves.

Chapter 3

The nurse–patient relationship – setting the scene

One of the most crucial aspects and under-rated elements of the nurse–patient relationship is the initial stage that ensures the therapeutic bond of that relationship. It would seem common sense that the first hello, a smile, that instant warm and friendly gesture be a natural and inherent part of the nurses' repertoire. Yet, for a whole host of reasons, not least of which might involve the increasing pressures upon nurses, this basic element is sometimes all too easily overlooked. The generation of warmth from one human being to another is a powerful gift and no amount of books on therapeutic communication can replace the experience of giving. There will, however, always be situations when someone in distress might not immediately respond to a caring approach and patience and perseverance, particularly initially, may be necessary. Consider the experience of trying to sort out a problem on the telephone with a company. By the time you have been passed from one person to the next, each asking you to explain yet again what the problem is, you are feeling pretty irate and uncooperative. If each person is distant and defensive, you can guarantee your irritability will escalate. However, if received by somebody with a warm and friendly voice who is helpful and understanding, even apologetic, then after your initial (understandable) fury, the effect is clear and you begin to calm down. This may take you by surprise and you may even feel a little deflated, yet, whatever your feelings, it often works. It is very difficult not to warm to this person. The same may be true of nursing. To keep your head when all around are losing theirs is vital. In the initial stages of any nurse–patient relationship or encounter, it is quite possible that you will be dealing with some very afraid, anxious, fraught, tired, uncertain or helpless individuals. In other words, individuals who may be perceived as 'difficult people'. It is your responsibility as a nurse to put your patients at ease and begin to sow the seeds of the therapeutic relationship.

Newell (1994) argues, 'lasting impressions are made from first meetings and the first moments of these meetings'. This is so very true. How many times have you met somebody for the first time and taken an instant like or dislike to that individual without knowing much, if anything about them? What is it that makes us like or dislike them? On initial contact it can only be the way they behave or present themselves (physically and psychologically). We particularly warm to people who appear to show a genuine interest in us and this is inevitably communicated through their verbal and non-verbal behaviour. The way they look at us, what they say, how they dress, how close they stand to us, their mannerisms, etc. How somebody 'sets the scene' with us, initially, colours the way we view future encounters with this individual. Sadly, one bad experience with another can wipe out numerous good experiences. Self-esteem is fragile and we all like to be liked.

Preparing the environment for a therapeutic and productive nurse–patient relationship consists of more than just physical bricks and mortar, but extends also to the nature, tone, atmosphere, context and experience of the overall relationship. The therapeutic environment includes both that which can be seen and touched and that which cannot. How we think and feel about ourselves, life and relationships at any given moment, or generally, will influence both our present and future relationships, particularly if we lack awareness. Newell (1994) likens both the initial and ongoing assessment phases of the nurse–patient relationship to a game of chess, 'in which the two participants come progressively to a greater understanding of each other'. Characteristically, he argues, 'the chess opening is extensively studied by players because it is crucial to what comes after'. It would seem we have much to learn from chess.

The therapeutic relationship is irrefutably more than just the sum of its parts and is far more complex than a distinct and entirely objective game. The course of any helping relationship tends to be recognized as a process and is largely considered in terms of four sequential parts or phases (Sundeen *et al.*, 1994). Each phase moves on from another and as such is developmental, as is life itself. In practice, the phases are mostly not mutually exclusive. Therefore, the environmental atmosphere of the nurse–patient relationship does not begin and end with the initial stages of the partnership, albeit crucial to them, but continues to be influenced by each stage and the focus and continued interactions within each stage.

The four phases identified by Sundeen *et al.* (1994) that the nurse and patient must work through, developed from the work of individuals such as Peplau (1952), are:

1. Pre-interaction phase
2. Orientation or introductory phase
3. Maintenance or working phase
4. Termination phase.

Pre-interaction phase

For the nurse, in many professional situations, relationships begin before the first face-to-face interaction with the client has even occurred. Preparations have to be made, possibly letters sent out, information about the client has to be accessed, telephone calls may be made, referrals discussed, I could go on. Communication about or even with the individual has begun before any meeting has actually taken place. In some circumstances, there may never in fact be a face-to-face meeting by the nature of need or your role as a health care professional. Information is often collated over a period of time and through a whole range of sources and an overall picture formed in both the minds of nurse and patient prior to any face-to-face communication. This picture, accurate or otherwise, is based on a combination of knowledge and past experiences, but is also introspective and may inevitably include a range of prejudices or negative attitudes about a variety of issues such as unemployment, mental illness, homosexuality, race, religion, gender, or practitioners themselves. Predetermined ideas may, of course, also be of a positive nature if individuals have had previously good experiences. Practitioners may or may not be aware of their own expectations and judgements or those of others. Therefore, recognition and self-awareness are important parts of the initial stages of an open and trusting relationship. First impressions are crucial and there is often no second chance to make an initial good impression.

Considerable time should be allocated to the careful collection of relevant material and information and sufficient consideration and preparation given to planning for the first or first few meetings. Remember you are communicating with your patient even before you have met him or her and setting the scene for future liaisons. As such the following issues should be taken into consideration whatever your setting of health care:

- Location
- Atmosphere
- Control
- Privacy
- Timing (Adapted from Sundeen *et al.*, 1994).

Location includes the accessibility and practicality of your chosen location. This is often outside the immediate control of practitioners themselves but a good knowledge of the 'whys' and 'wherefores' with regard to getting to the hospital or clinic and so forth is useful. The provision of directions (verbal or written), information about availability of transport and making the necessary arrangements if appropriate, timetables and a good understanding of your patient's individual needs can promote confidence in the system.

Some patients will have no problem making their own way, while others will struggle or fail to attend due to impracticalities. This problem commonly contributes to the rising number of inappropriate medical emergency admissions (Duxbury, 1999b). It is important the nurse is aware of these pre-interaction issues. With regard to the nursing environment itself within the location, the nurse has far more control and one may wish to consider the arrangement of the immediate environment such as furniture and decor. This, in turn can create a relaxed and/or professional atmosphere.

Atmosphere refers to both physical and psychological presence. Initial and subsequent meetings and interactions with patients will usually be held in the same place. This might be the patient's bed-space area, a quiet corner of the unit, a specific room, or the nurse's office. Whatever the setting, it is your aim to try to create as relaxing and comfortable an atmosphere as possible. For instance, furniture can create barriers or facilitate sharing. It is a fairly well accepted fact today that it is not useful to place desks between yourself and your patient (Arnold and Boggs, 1995). Arrange what furniture you can to promote equality. Chairs need to be close enough to provide support and touch if necessary, but not too close that an individual's space is invaded (Egan, 1998). Be adaptable, chairs are mostly not fixed to the floor, move in and out as necessary. Remember to watch for verbal and non-verbal cues. Lighting can also be effective, bright lights can exacerbate tension. Background music may be a valuable source of relaxation. It is easy to lose sight of individual control when working for large organizations. Adaptation of the immediate environment can be beneficial to the patient. This does not necessarily mean insisting upon new and purpose-built offices, but may be the provision of minor and subtle changes to existing environments. Above all, initial meetings and the creation of a welcoming and warm atmosphere can be the most essential tool in any nurse's communication kit. This has much to do with our presentation of self as warm, open, listening and caring, but also has a great deal to do with the last three issues of the pre-interaction phase – control, privacy and timing. Initial preparations for meetings with clients should include ensuring that we are ready to greet them on their arrival. This is possible in the case of emergency admissions if sufficient staffing levels and a state of readiness are secured. Whatever the context, the allocation of privacy both in physical settings and by promoting trust in how relationships are conducted can facilitate good presentation (Farrell and Gray, 1992). Interruptions, in particular, must be reduced to a minimum and a nurse allocated the necessary amount of time and space prior to the meeting. The necessary control over all these issues in advance is crucial to a stress-free initial consultation for both nurse and patient. This in turn will inspire confidence and prepare the way for greater therapeutic communication.

The ward environment, in particular, can be an extremely busy place and may seem disorganized and chaotic to the newly admitted patient. There is nothing worse than turning up on a ward or for an appointment only to find there is no record of you and that nobody is expecting you. I bet you can think of at least one occasion when this has been the case. Good preparation and organizational skills in this initial pre-interaction can reduce the risk of such problems arising. Taking care of what may seem to be minor, even non-nurse related preparations could smooth the way for better nurse–patient relations in the long term. This, in turn, may lessen the incidence of uncooperative, difficult patients based on the underlying anxiety associated with hospitalization and/or health care and, particularly, a loss of confidence in staff from the start.

Accepting that the progress of the nurse–patient relationship is on a continuum with a very important beginning and end phase is vital (Newell, 1994). Relationships do not just happen, one has to work at them, whatever the relationship, in order to make them work. While both nurse and patient have equally important parts and responsibilities, the nurse can be a key player in working through the phases of this relationship and in guiding the patients over the many hurdles he or she may have to face. The next important phase that is an extension of the pre-interaction phase and necessary preparation is the introductory phase, also commonly referred to as the orientation phase (Peplau, 1952; Newell, 1994).

Introductory phase

Having prepared for and paved the way for the initial encounter, the first meeting between the nurse and client sets the scene for the rest of the relationship. The intimate relationships formed in health are by nature and context unusual ones and often intimacy is initiated very early on, missing out the usual steps for the development of such relationships. Often this intimacy of both a physical and resulting psychological nature is unavoidable. However, the orientation phase of the partnership can do much to ease the path for all involved.

Initial meetings with patients may not always be planned or prepared for in ways I have suggested earlier. The way you engage in contact with a particular patient may vary enormously from day to day and combine an array of irregularities in balance, power and need. Consider the following of how contact with a patient may start:

1. The patient is sick; the nurse is healthy.
2. The patient is needy; the nurse can attempt to fulfil the need.
3. The patient may have only the nurse to relate to; the nurse has other patients and colleagues to relate to if he or she needs time out. The nurse can also go home at the end of the day. Some patients cannot.
4. The patient is dependent; the nurse has power.
5. The patient may be lying down; the nurse is standing over him or her.
6. The patient may have needs of intimate bodily care, and the nurse, a stranger, gives it without question or address about the level or phase of the relationship.

This list adapted from the work of Tschudin (1993) makes it quite clear that the relationship between a nurse and patient can be basically very imbalanced. Salvage (1990) argues that we are beginning to enter a new era whereby the focus of the nurse–patient relationship is that of partnership. Partnership that has to be worked on, established and negotiated. This is one of the major objectives of phase two; the introductory phase.

The establishment of expectations, needs, roles and the way forward are priorities of this very early stage. As such the following factors must be taken into consideration and handled in such a way as to set the scene for a trusting and mutual relationship.

Introductions

This involves not only the elementary niceties of the warm smile, the handshake and the 'hello my name is... and I am your helper, primary nurse, named nurse or therapist, which are vitally important in their own right, but also the rudiments of where to sit, why you are meeting, how this has come about and the objectives of the first meeting. The introduction is also a part of the process that allows patients to settle into a new setting, find their bearings, relax a little and get to know you before tackling more complex issues. The first meeting should not be heavy. Patience is crucial when easing clients into this new relationship, time permitting, as the basis for trust and rapport is established. The introduction may just involve a few brief minutes with a new patient while being admitted and orientation to their new environment, or may be a more formal part of a lengthier, introductory meeting. Both formats have their part to play and can be effective if planned for.

The contract

The next objective of this initial encounter will involve the establishment of a contract to identify ground rules and negotiate roles in light of explored expectations, ability and experience (Lorig, 1992). Once again, depending upon the setting and chosen approach, this may be formal or otherwise. Whatever the format, at the end of initial discussions, expectations must be clearly defined, understood and agreed to. This may be a lengthy process and require some degree of patience and negotiation. Patients come to health care settings with all sorts of preconceived ideas, some of which may be accurate, some of which may be misguided.

A contract serves to describe the nature and content of the relationship and as mentioned involves the process of negotiation between you and your patient. For instance, you may want to discuss and establish a whole range of issues such as how to address each other (i.e. first names), where and how often you will meet, purpose of your interactions (short-term goals can be set and evaluated), who will be involved in care, privacy and confidentiality, who to address if need be, punctuality and attendance (if appropriate), record keeping and care plans, expected length of treatment therapy, visiting times, smoking, cancellation, discharge and any other issues that might need clarification in order to assist the smooth running of the relationship and orientation to norms. Social norms and boundaries are an integral part of life and can promote a feeling of safety in a supportive but flexible atmosphere. The key to successful contracts is that they are mutually agreed and owned by both participants. They are not contracts made by the nurse for the patient to follow, as this will only lead to mistrust, lack of relevance to the individual and inevitable non-compliance (a difficult patient behaviour) (Cameron and Gregor, 1987). Contracts must be thrashed out between nurse and patient until accepted goals are agreed upon. This may require a little give and take, through the exploration of expectations, needs, viewpoints and shared knowledge. Both nurse and patient must adhere to them in order for them to work effectively. A whole initial session may be spent on 'contracting' but will be time well spent, the outcome of which will ensure clarification of the roles of the nurse and patient in this new founded relationship.

A practical formula for making a contract

1. First decide what you are hoping to accomplish as patients will be looking for guidance from you.
2. Arrange a meeting with the patient and explore with them what *they* hope to achieve. Start from the broad and work down to measurable specifics, e.g. meditate for 20 minutes three times a week.
3. Negotiate your expectations and the patients' expectations and discuss alternatives as necessary.
4. Make a concrete plan which should contain the following elements:
   (a) Exactly *what* the patient will do
   (b) When they will do this – time span. *Do not* be over-ambitious.
   (c) How often will they do this? e.g. twice a week, five minutes per day, etc.
   (d) Any active part you might play.
5. Identify rewards for each target met. They must be chosen by the patient if they are to be meaningful and effective. Targets and rewards are best if set on a short-term, regular basis. If goals are too long term, they become inept.
6. Check the validity of the contract. Ask the patient on a scale of 0–100 (0 being totally unsure and 100 being absolutely sure), how certain they are that they will adhere to the contract. If they answer 70+ then it will probably be successful (Lorig, 1992). If they answer less than 70, then go back over points 1–5 and rethink accordingly.
7. Once agreed, formally write out the contract, agree a review date and both parties sign it.

Roles of the nurse–client relationship

Orientation of the client will occur or at least should occur if the nurse is communicating effectively throughout the course of the nursing relationship. The initial interview is an essential starting point. Orientation is assisted by a full exploration and explanation of the nurse–patient process and should contain the following important components advocated by Newell (1994):

- A description of the nurse's perceived initial formulation of the client's difficulties.
- A general description of the rationale underlying the nurse's/doctor's proposed interventions for the problem.
- Specific examples of what is likely to be expected of the client. For instance, to meet at set times, take medication, learn about wound care, attend set therapy settings and so on, depending upon problem area(s).
- Specific examples of what the client can expect of the nurse, for instance, demonstration, doing for, support, teaching, the provision of information, assisting and so on depending upon level of need.
- A discussion in relation to prognosis and outcome, if known.
- Emphasis upon negotiation and recognition that both nurse and patient have rights in this process.
- Ongoing assessment and evaluation to monitor progress in relation to health and effectiveness of working relationship.

Objectives such as these can only be met if the right environment is encouraged through both the pre-interaction and introductory phase. Peplau (1994) argues that the initial meeting is crucial in setting the correct pattern for future nurse–patient interaction, the desirable pattern being one, in which the patient does most of the talking and the nurse listens, intermittently addressing a question about whatever the patient has just said. This in turn, initially at least, facilitates the exploration of problems and concerns as seen from the patient's perspective, encouraged with the use of active listening and attending skills, and paves the way for the nurse to then offer his or her perspective. The two perspectives must then be married. In the situation of a new patient, despite the likelihood that the newcomer and nurse are both well intentioned, there can be mismatches. This arises often indirectly from the imbalance between presuppositions of the patient and the stock of knowledge of the nurse which can lead to each viewing the other as prejudiced or unresponsive (Ashworth *et al.*, 1992). Information sharing and negotiation is therefore essential in rectifying this imbalance in the introductory phase.

Some practitioners are fairly new to or feel less experienced in early preparatory and initial interviewing skills. Peplau (1994) advocates that there are some basic guidelines which can build confidence in therapeutic communication and develop practitioner techniques. They include the following points:

1. Remember that patients do not die from interviews. They have many ways to manage any possible stress effects from the interview and are very likely to use these relief behaviours. What is likely to happen, however, is that they will gain some beneficial effect from your sustained interest in them and their increased feeling of self-worth.

2. Make your mistakes openly, then examine and rectify them. This will promote trust. After your initial meeting, review your notes, critique your verbal content and amend your approach at the next meeting. Use your mistakes to learn from. This is a useful rule of thumb for all practitioners irrespective of level of experience and skill.

3. Prior to each encounter, check your expectations. Go into communications with realistic expectations and an open mind. This will help manage your own anxiety and self-worth.

4. It is possible that initially you will feel awkward and uncomfortable while gaining experience. Remember the first bath or injection you gave. Interviewing and learning to communicate therapeutically can have the same 'newness' and unfamiliarity about it. You will survive. The second meeting or encounter may feel easier.

5. Take notice of responses evoked in you by the patients in initial meetings. Write them down as soon as possible after the interview. These are clues to intentions and the general interpersonal patterns of the patient.

6. In addition, I would suggest that you always remember that communication is a two-way process (Peel, 1995). While as a health care practitioner you have to take responsibility for your professional conduct and share of the partnership (UKCC, 1992), patients too must own their own behaviour. The onus is upon you to lead the way, orientate and encourage a relationship, which in turn facilitates communication and enables the patient to return to an optimum level of well-being. However, if patients present behaviour that is 'difficult', they must accept their part to play when things are not working out. Examine your behaviour and choice of approach and learn from it but do not beat yourself up about limited progress. Work through it.

Relationships are rarely plain sailing particularly given the difficulties and stresses associated with a need for health care. The supportive foundations of the therapeutic relationship are established in the earlier two phases and provide a solid base on which to 'work through' the inevitable problems that nurse–patient relationships will encounter. As such, the majority of the work and interventions will materialize in the third phase of this relationship, aptly named the working phase.

Working phase

Forchuk (1994) proposes that as many as one in three patients are discharged from hospital or transferred while still in Peplau's orientation phase of the nurse–patient relationship. This implies that a large group of clients never reach this working phase and as a result are discharged or transferred without ever establishing any degree of trust with their nurses or before identifying problems to be worked on within their hospitalization. This not only highlights the importance of and possibly lengthy process of the orientation phase, which may take several meetings to work through, but also raises concerns about the nurse's ability to move patients through this phase successfully to work on problems.

The working phase described by both Peplau (1952) and later Sundeen *et al.* (1994) involves the identification and utilization of communication strategies and nursing interventions that are needed for problem resolution and the continued enhancement of self-concept. It is expected by this stage that any atmosphere of trust and rapport will have been initiated, making it easier for the patient to discuss deeper more difficult issues and to experiment with new roles and actions in a safe environment.

It is a large part of the nurse's responsibility to do all he or she can during this phase to enable this to happen. As suggested by the title, the working phase requires input and labour from both the nurse and patient, the emphasis being mutuality and client autonomy. This involves facilitating a careful balance between the client's need for protection and his or her equally important need for self-determination and independence. Clients' perceptions of their health requirements need to be heard and understood. They need to feel they have had some degree of control in their care and played a sufficiently vital part (Arnold and Bogg, 1995), particularly as in many instances, this self-sufficiency will need to be continued while recovering.

A structured overview of this phase would involve:

- Defining the problem
- Pacing progress

- Developing realistic goals which are clear and specific
- Planning and evaluating possible solutions with client
- Implementing a plan
- Exploring and handling resistance
- Ongoing evaluation
- Referral if appropriate
- Recognition of timing for the termination phase (Adapted from Arnold and Boggs, 1995).

The emphasis upon responsibility for the various steps will shift and alternate depending upon progress. The combination of steps may seem familiar as they clearly resemble the stages of the nursing process (McFarlane and Castledine, 1982). As such the mechanics of each step will not be dealt with in this text but can be found within the realms of other written material on the nursing process.

The termination phase will be dealt with separately in the final chapter.

Having explored basic frameworks that can assist practitioners in their role, the practical interventions necessary for the facilitation of therapeutic communication and the management of difficult patients will now be addressed as the working phase of the nurse–patient relationship, in the following chapter. The following encompasses a specific set of strategies to be used as a reference for the recognized difficulties nurses and health care workers encounter in the health care field, with some suggested practical solutions based on Heron (1990), largely, and others in this field.

Chapter 4

Managing the difficult patient – strategies and intervention for protective behaviours

Protective behaviours – withdrawal and passivity

For the purpose of this book, patient behaviours and states have been categorized into four main areas: withdrawn, passive, challenging and confrontational patients. Each type of difficult patient can then be further grouped into two larger forms of patient behaviour termed protective and defensive behaviours. This can be seen more clearly in Figure 4.1.

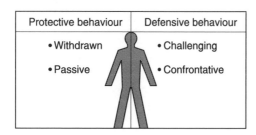

Protective behaviour	Defensive behaviour
• Withdrawn	• Challenging
• Passive	• Confrontative

Figure 4.1 Protective and defensive patient behaviours

Protective behaviours

Protective behaviours are common in health care and may be employed by patients knowingly or unconsciously. They are those behaviours that patients may exhibit while trying literally to 'protect' themselves from the reality or pain of what is facing them whilst ill. Withdrawal and passivity are common features of protective behaviours seen in patients. Non-compliance is possibly one of the most common problems encountered in this patient group and is estimated to affect 30–70% of nurse–patient encounters (Lorig, 1992). While patients present with such behaviours for a variety of reasons, there is often an underlying need not to get involved actively in their care. This may be because they are trying to resist or deny what is happening to them, do not want to get involved or do not know how to. As such, these patients frequently have very specific needs that respond well to the specific nursing skills of facilitation. An authoritarian approach may also be warranted in the early stages of the nurse–patient relationship, but the goal is to enable the individual.

Defensive behaviours, on the other hand, are more commonly seen as hostility by challenging and confrontational patients, although at times this hostility may, in fact, be quite subtle. In contrast to protective behaviours, defensive behaviours warrant a facilitative approach in the initial stage of the nurse–patient relationship, while authoritative skills are frequently required as the relationship and behaviours progress. Defensive behaviours and resulting approaches are dealt with separately in greater detail in Chapter 5.

It is not the intention of the author to suggest that patients can always be neatly categorized in this way without exception. This format is purely for convenience and accessibility to the reader. While it has been recognized for some time that the use of patient labels can be detrimental to the nurse–patient relationship (Illich, 1990), diagnostic labels such as the 'aggressive patient' continue to be used (Miller, 1990). Hadfield-Law (1998) suggests that practitioners are not immune to prejudice and argues 'perhaps it is not the prejudice itself that needs to be addressed but our awareness'.

The following extract from a US news item is a useful example:

> Within 3 minutes of entering the courtroom, a prospective juror told the judge he couldn't be on the jury because he'd seen the defendant and knew he was guilty. The judge noted where he was pointing and told him the man he thought was the defendant was the prosecuting attorney.
>
> (Cited in Hadfield-Law, 1998.)

Clients can, in fact, demonstrate a whole array of behaviours at any one time or over a period of time that may well cross the boundaries of the 'types' identified above. Patients are individuals and must be treated as such; however, as every individual situation cannot be addressed in a generalist book of this nature, commonalities have to be relied upon. Helping strategies such as those outlined in the work of Heron (1990) can also be easily categorized. Each category recommended by Heron is not self-limiting and strategies can be mixed and matched, chosen or ignored. For instance, strategies recommended specifically for one type of client can be cross-fertilized and used for a variety of problems, type of patient or client setting. It is for the practitioner and patient to determine, either alone or together, in light of explored perceptions and needs, the most appropriate avenues to take and at the most appropriate time. The following approaches and suggested interventions are guidelines only and not intended to be a dogma nor expected to be so. There is, however, a need for practicalities and the development of a range of skill-based solutions from which the practitioner may choose when caring for 'difficult clients'. Avoidance, professional withdrawal and defensive approaches are non-therapeutic and unproductive, while the principles of therapeutic communication have much to offer (Smith and Hart, 1994).

Throughout the following two chapters there will be a range of familiar interventions, some that may seem difficult to achieve and others that will be viewed as basic common sense. The material used is drawn from a variety of sources and experiences and presented in a way that is accessible, applicable, practical and relevant to issues related to difficult patients, their behaviour and the promotion of effective communication in the health care setting. The approach advocated encourages the examination of practice and exploration of the needs of vulnerable patients. This is particularly important given the increasing level of patient dissatisfaction with health care (Rogers *et al.*, 1993) and the rising concern from practitioners relating to difficult patients (Hadfield-Law, 1998).

Getting to know patients and their unique experience, while recognizing the existence of factors common to all individuals, is crucial to the overall approach in this book.

Some nurses assume they know patients based on limited data, stereotypes regarding age, social class or diagnostic group, and this is especially true when dealing with difficult patients (Stockwell, 1984). Getting to know a patient means talking to and with that person, involves investigation, purpose, accurate listening and a goal-related framework. These elements are the building blocks necessary for the development of therapeutic communication (Arnold and Boggs, 1995) that allow the nurse and patient to grow, change, and become human as a consequence (Peplau, 1994). This is your aim irrespective of how a patient presents. Whether a withdrawn, passive, challenging or confrontational patient, the helper's role is to determine how to help and facilitate progress. Every patient has a need, every need is a challenge and every encounter between nurse and patient has the potential for increasingly positive outcomes.

Table 4.1 Factors which may contribute to difficult behaviour

Protective behaviour

Withdrawal	*Passivity*
• Pain	• Cultural influences
• Fear	• Patient rules historically
• Lack of sleep/rest	• Personality – introverted
• Non-compliance	• Communication difficulties
• Loneliness	– Language barriers
• Uncertainty	– Lack of understanding
• Despair	– Results of physical problems due to illness
• Low motivation	– Impaired cognition
	– Effects of medication
	– Practitioner dominance

Defensive behaviour

Challenge	*Confrontation*
Attention-needing behaviour:	• Anger
• Interfering	• Frustration
• Over-involvement	• Lack of control
• Demanding	• Response to confrontation/aggression
• Sexually explicit	• Intoxication
• Insecurity	

Strategies for intervention and related issues when caring for withdrawn and passive patients

To feel alone is an experience common to most at some point throughout life's course. To withdraw can be a protective behaviour in response to a perceived threat. The stress of everyday life reveals itself in many ways and the stress of illness, coupled with the uncertainty of hospitalization, will inevitably take its toll on even the strongest and hardiest of personalities. Everybody reacts to stress and strain differently (Ogden, 1998). For some, becoming withdrawn and distant is a natural response, yet for others, passivity can be interpreted by the health care worker as hostility, uncooperativeness, lack of interest and generally as 'difficult behaviour'. With any presenting behaviour, one must strive to see what lies beyond the exterior and look for answers in order to be able to understand more objectively and help more effectively. Often the subjectivity of what we see and feel inhibits our ability to care. It is important to recognize and accept such feelings in order to communicate therapeutically. This is commonly referred to as self-awareness (Kagan and Evans, 1995).

Stress is perceived in different ways by different people. It may be seen as an external factor, a stressor, or manifest in how we feel (Ogden, 1998). When it becomes a problem, how it is dealt with is also unique to the individual. For instance, coping may involve a drink in the pub at the end of the day, a hot bath, a moan to a good friend, a game of squash and so on. It is only when stress overwhelms or when a variety of stressors occur at any one given time, particularly when resources and support are limited, that coping becomes problematic and may become maladaptive. For example, drinking excessively, ignoring what is happening or withdrawal. Powell and Enright (1993) argue there are three important components for understanding an individual's personal model of stress. They are:

1. The idea that demands tax our system in some way (the external view).
2. The idea that there is some form of appraisal or perception of threat which in turn affects our response.

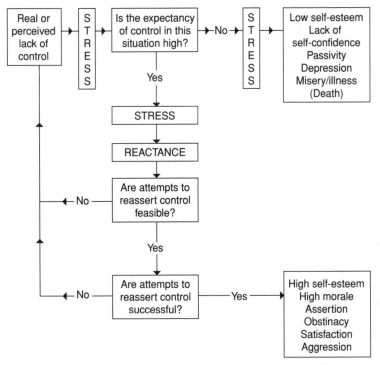

Figure 4.2 Consequences of real and perceived lack of control for self-esteem. Reproduced with permission of Stanley Thornes Publishers Ltd from *Professional Interpersonal Skills for Nurses*, Kagan and Evans, 1995.

3. The importance of the response upon that system – what the behaviour is and how it affects the individual (the internal view).

The basic skills and principles mentioned in preceding chapters can facilitate greater understanding of the patient's experience, how they perceive their situation and their response. In addition, what the threats are, what they mean and how they are coped with are important considerations. Withdrawal may only be one form of behaviour that reveals a level of stress unacceptable to the individual.

Inevitably, people have and develop preferred or familiar styles of dealing with conflict. Some of these are more constructive than others.

Maddux (1988) suggests four common ways of resolving conflict, some which are adaptive and some less so:

• Avoidance
• Accommodation
• Win/lose/compromise
• Problem solving.

Each differs in terms of assertiveness and cooperation as seen below (Figure 4.3).

Some patients may use a mixture of styles at various points on the grid and strategies will vary according to the situation and people involved. Nurses have an important part to play in how the individual may react. The most constructive strategies will be

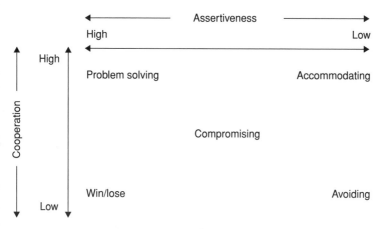

Figure 4.3 Methods of conflict resolution in terms of assertiveness and cooperation (from Kagan and Evans, 1995)

those that are both high in cooperation and assertiveness which is important for patient participation and autonomy (Brearley, 1990). The least constructive are those that are low in cooperation and low in assertiveness. In this instance, withdrawal, which may indicate avoidance, is the problem. Avoidance and/or denial of the problem often drive withdrawal behaviours (Miller, 1990).

It is important throughout this and the following chapters to accept that the basic principles and skills addressed in previous chapters are an integral and important part of all strategies discussed specifically, and for the overall presenting behaviours of all difficult patients. They will, therefore, not be revisited again when discussing strategies for each type of patient. This would only result in repetition. It is also important to note that, although individual types of intervention categories (Heron, 1990) are highlighted for each 'difficult patient' group where deemed to be particularly useful, this does not exclude the use of other categories. There will, inevitably, be frequent overlaps between categories and the need for a combination of approaches or for changing an approach if felt to be necessary. The use of some categories of intervention, such as supportive interventions, will be required for all patients but to varying levels dependent upon

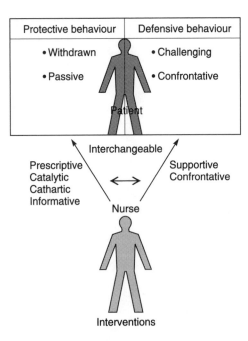

Figure 4.4 An overview of patient behaviours and advocated strategies

need(s) and the duration of hospitalization. While Heron's categories are emphasized, the author has been selective in the interventions chosen for inclusion in a nursing context and in the incorporation of additional strategies under relevant headings.

In summary, Heron's framework has been adapted to suit the needs of the hospital health care setting and recommended strategies, both included and excluded as deemed appropriate.

Strategies for caring for the withdrawn or passive patient

Underlying avoidance and possible denial of perceived threats may be driving the behaviour of withdrawn and passive patients. With this in mind, four specific categories of intervention will be particularly important for such individuals. They are:

- Prescriptive
- Cathartic
- Catalytic
- Informative (From Heron, 1990).

The withdrawn and passive patient needs the skills of effective facilitation and as such, facilitative categories are ideal. Prescription, while an authoritative approach, can be valuable initially, followed with progressive facilitation.

Prescriptive interventions

There are two essential issues to consider when opting to use a prescriptive approach:

- How to prescribe – prescription is a term commonly associated with medicine; the term, however, has much more to offer than that. For instance, prescription may be direct or in consultation with a patient. It may involve the prescription of a course of action, a change in thinking, some self-directed work or actual treatment. It is very much an integral part of any nursing role and can be used as a valuable building block.
- Whether to prescribe at all – a patient may or may not be ready or able to make decisions about his or her care, ability or behaviour, without assistance. This is a fundamental issue for all practitioners particularly when deliberating what, when and how best to intervene based on the level of patient need.

There will inevitably be times when patients are not in a position to make choices for themselves whether due to physical, psychological or social incapacity. As such, the nurse's prescriptive role at that point will largely be to prescribe a direct course of action and in some instances to carry out this action on behalf of the patient until the individual is able to function independently (Heron, 1990).

Forms of prescription

When prescribing, there are various ways this can be done:

1. *Directive prescription* – the nurse may advise, propose, recommend, suggest and request certain behaviours from the patient without directly seeking the client's opinion or agreement about the proposed behaviour. This may be acceptable in a range of situations such as the unconscious patient, in an emergency situation or when detaining patients under the Mental Health Act (Department of Health, 1983). Heron (1990) advocates, of course, it is essential that the nurse is open to dissent from the patient and that patients are not forced to comply when out of the boundaries of the above, even if you know it is crucial they follow your prescription. Hence there is a directive prescription continuum ranging from the mild to the strong type of direction given (Heron, 1990).

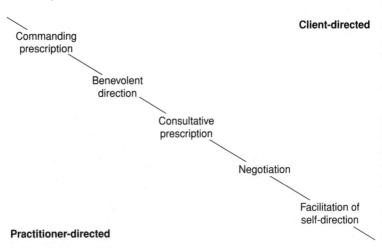

Figure 4.5 Continuum: the prescriptive–catalytic gradient (from Heron, 1990). Reprinted by permission of Sage Publications Ltd.

It is helpful to make use of this framework and to inform the patient, where appropriate, from which part of the continuum you are working. This may have much to do with their perceptions of your role and status and as such should not be abused.

2. *Consultative prescription* – this intervention relies more heavily upon consultation with the patient and an exploration of their views about options available. While consultation is sought, this still remains a largely authoritative approach and it is assumed that within the relationship the nurse, in light of the patient's beliefs, will still make the ultimate decision. Patients tend to view health practitioners as experts with the relevant knowledge and expertise to make the right prescriptions (Luker and Waterworth, 1990). However, the art of consultation coupled with explanation is advocated as the way forward (Brearley, 1990).

3. *Action research prescription* – here it is proposed that patients try out new behaviours experimentally, with a view to this course of action being pursued in the future, if successful. In many ways, it resembles a 'trial and error' approach and also requires consultation and discussion with the patient. Health care today is complex and increasingly there are limited answers to expanding questions. A variety of interventions commonly have to be explored and evaluated until the most fitting strategy is found. Demanding and confrontational patients may feel uncertain about their care or future and may benefit from this approach on an experimental basis to give them some direction. In order to prescribe in this way, practitioners must be honest about their certainty, or lack of it, relating to the interventions prescribed. This will promote a degree of trust and avoid further confrontation.

4. *Homework prescription* – homework can be a very useful part of information giving and a way of reviewing a patient's understanding of the information given (Lorig, 1992). While requiring some level of cooperation, it is largely a prescriptive category whereby patients are asked to comply or even told what to do and what is required to proceed. Homework often relates to where a patient is and the treatment strategy employed. It must not be aimed too high or too soon. Again, although directive, it can be facilitative in that it gives direction and requires some degree of involvement/control. This is particularly crucial when caring for patients who present as challenging or confrontational. Often, the underlying lack of control is an issue coupled with feelings of neglect. Ongoing

interventions that incorporate planning, involvement, timing and above all input of time from practitioners, are paramount when caring for difficult patients.

5. *Demonstrative prescription* – the input of patience and time with a patient can promote feelings of worth and underpins the success of this strategy. When wanting patients to adopt certain behaviours necessary for their well-being, demonstration is a useful tool. Prescription is achieved by directly showing a patient what you want them to do or by more subtly role modelling a proposed behaviour. Like many other forms of prescription, this approach may be directive or consultative but requires some level of client autonomy. Once given a demonstration and opportunities for supervised rehearsal, the patient is then required to go off and practise alone. The provision of written material to support the main points of the demonstration can be a useful aide memoire (Reece and Walker, 1997).

6. *Follow the leader prescription* – this may be incorporated into demonstration or may indeed stand alone as an approach. The nurse leads the way, not merely by demonstration, but by doing the targeted behaviour for real with the client. Both nurse and patient keep a personal diary of outcomes. This may only be appropriate for certain individuals and in certain situations. It may be particularly useful in health promotion and education settings where weight loss or cessation of smoking is necessary, or when working with withdrawn and passive patients who may need you to take the lead, by example, to encourage and inspire.

7. *Validating prescription* – this involves the recommendation of a particular course of action by the nurse. The patient is then encouraged to participate by affirming their worth, your belief in them and their ability to succeed. For instance, 'I know you can do this Jenny'. In this way individual and special attributes and strengths are acknowledged and emphasized. Withdrawn and passive patients may have underlying feelings of low self-esteem or lack of confidence and as such, this approach can be very therapeutic.

8. *Retrospective prescription* – this technique requires examination of past behaviours and outcomes. This is a useful approach when working with patients who have had similar problems before and who have been either successful or unsuccessful in managing them. If unsuccessful previously, patients can learn from this experience; conversely, when successful, strength can be utilized and built upon. A diary

may be a useful tool for this approach, encouraging reflection upon progress or lack of it (Palmer *et al.*, 1994).

9. *Paradoxical prescription* – this and the remaining two strategies must be used sensitively and by practitioners with some degree of experience, understanding and/or supervision. Above all, the intentions of the nurse must be to help the client make progress. The nurse endeavours to propose that, although a course of action is recommended, it is believed that the patient will be unable to carry it out successfully. This is not meant to be disrespectful, but is intended to spur the patient into action. It may remotivate the passive or withdrawn individual. It is a sort of 'I'll show him or her' response that is hoped for and even if driven by annoyance, as opposed to inspiration, can be both practical and acceptable. Obviously, when choosing to use such a strategy, it must be clearly identified and the underlying philosophy documented. The nurse must feel confident in using the approach and be prepared for possible unwanted feedback. If it does not produce the desired effect, it is crucial the nurse enlightens the patient as to what he or she was hoping to achieve. Relatives and significant others must also be informed and a consistent team approach advocated.

10. *Contradictory prescription* – in this approach the patient is prescribed or informed of two opposing courses of action. For instance, while suggesting that a patient should stay in bed all day, an explanation is given that thrombus can be caused by immobility. It is anticipated that when faced with this conflicting dilemma, the patient will opt for the most sensible (desirable) behaviour, which in this instance would be to mobilize, or find a compromise. This approach is based on the principles of cognitive therapy. It is assumed that individuals will not tolerate something called 'cognitive dissonance' (conflicting ideas) and will take some course of action to relieve the discomfort felt (Newell, 1994).

11. *Counter-dependent prescription* – finally, this form of prescription can be adopted. This strategy is based upon basic assumptions about the nature of human behaviour. It is commonly recognized that if you ask some people to do something and, particularly, if you insist on action, they will often do the opposite. In many instances, we like to exercise our own independence and feel uncomfortable being told what to do. This may be true of some patients on admission to hospital who will act out of character if anxious or afraid. If previous strategies have failed, this can be a useful approach.

Example 1

Counter-dependent prescription can be effective for patients who cannot sleep. For instance, if a specific request is made to the patient that they must stay awake all night, inevitably, in the majority of cases, they will want to sleep.

Example 2

When working with a passive or withdrawn patient, instruct them to increase their passivity in the hope that they will want to, in turn, do the opposite and become more directly involved. This may warrant a statement such as 'given that you do not want to be involved in your care, I will not give you any more information and will just go ahead and treat you'. Response to this approach can be surprising and patients may become more inquisitive and ask more questions.

Overall, prescription is far more complex than just telling somebody what to do and how to lead their life, which is commonly unsuccessful as a strategy in isolation. Prescription can be seen on a graded continuum, the ultimate aim being to enable patients to become more self-sufficient. Prescription, therefore, may be a useful and valid tool at the start of a patient's admission or first contact with health care services, but should not be seen as a means in itself. It is part of an ongoing process and may need to be revisited on many occasions in the patient's experience, during any setbacks or the development of new problems.

Cathartic interventions

In order to address the problem(s) the withdrawn or passive patient may be experiencing, it is first necessary to help clients express any feelings and undischarged distress that is disabling or distorting their behaviour. This is the aim of catharsis – to facilitate expression of emotion in a supportive way.

There are different sorts of stress clients may need to work on. Firstly, there may be distress, including physical tension, pain, anger, fear, anxiety, grief, embarrassment and/or any combination of the range of human emotion that one can experience. Secondly, the cause of the distress, the stressor, may warrant attention. The nurse can facilitate expression of a variety of feelings by creating the right sort of therapeutic environment. This can be promoted using the following skills and strategies:

The nurse's first responsibility is to create a warm and accepting atmosphere conducive to trust and exploration of the patient's distress. This can often be achieved using the basic skills of active listening and empathy as discussed in Chapter 2. Exploration can also be encouraged using a variety of open and closed questions and the timely use of silence.

Questions and the way they are used can be very important. The way a question is asked in part determines how well it is received and its effectiveness (Kagan and Evans, 1995). 'Different situations coupled with *the purpose* of questioning, determine which style is most appropriate' (Dillon, 1990) and as such most useful.

There are two distinct types of questions, which are commonly referred to as open and closed questions (Burnard, 1989; Arnold and Boggs, 1995). Closed questions are those that limit the possibilities of reply and are often used to collect specific information. They frequently invite yes/no or one-worded answers and do not generally open up the conversation, particularly with a withdrawn patient. Conversely, closed questions may be valuable initially in making some contact as they are far less threatening. For instance, 'does it hurt you?' or 'you feel sad don't you?'. Open questions, on the other hand, invite conversation if used with confidence and allow freedom of response. For example, 'how do you feel?', 'what is worrying you?', 'tell me a little more'. However, when using open questions, the practitioner must feel able to encourage short periods of silence in order to allow sufficient time for response. This is not an easy skill, and in addition to cathartic techniques generally, is one area that health care workers are least comfortable with (Burnard and Morrison, 1991). Withdrawn patients who feel threatened and in a state of distress will commonly need additional time and patience from nurses before responding. They may be struggling to find the words, find it difficult to express what they are thinking or feeling or just simply not know what is happening to them and withdraw as a result.

Patience is crucial. Several short visits to patients may be necessary in order to build up a level of rapport.

The use of encouraging verbal prompts to facilitate expression can be valuable. For instance, 'this is difficult for you I know' or 'it's okay, take your time'. Strategies of this kind coupled with non-verbal 'small rewards' such as an encouraging smile, intermittent eye contact or the nod of a head when listening are both supportive and reassuring. Patients need to know we are interested and ready to listen. To promote a degree of confidence this must be reflected both verbally and non-verbally by the practitioner (Nelson-Jones, 1994).

Sitting in close proximity to patients and at a similar level which, in turn, facilitates the use of touch as deemed appropriate, is a useful approach. This may involve simply reaching out to touch the patient's arm in a supportive way or may involve more intimate contact such as an embrace when a client begins to express emotion (Heron, 1990). The use of advanced empathy can facilitate recognition of when it is okay and when it is not okay to invade a patient's personal space. In this way signals of resistance from a patient such as drawing back must be respected and it is important for the nurse to withdraw a little if this is the case (Egan, 1998).

Some patients find it exceptionally difficult to open up to anybody, let alone professionals whom they have only known for a short time. This is hardly surprising as many people only talk openly to those closest to them. Nurses are frequently in the unusual position of being with individuals who are in turmoil or pain. It is important, therefore, to use sensitivity to assist patients to open up gradually.

Having gained the initial confidence of a patient, the following three-stage approach can be useful in promoting and encouraging further catharsis (Heron, 1990):

(a) From analysis to incident – here, if a patient appears silently preoccupied with a current difficulty or problem, they can be prompted to try to describe in a concrete way, specific examples of how they are feeling or the traumatic event that is worrying them. For some patients, there may be several issues. Often one is enough to tackle at any given time, and by asking the patient to 'describe what is worrying them the most', problems can be prioritized and tackled in stages.

(b) Encourage a more literal description – next, ask the patient not just to offer an outline of what has happened or is happening, but to describe the traumatic experience in literal detail, recalling vivid sights, sounds, smells, thoughts and what people said and did. Heron (1990) argues 'distress is lodged in imagery of all kinds' and can be drawn up by using this technique. To recall sensory experiences that are associated with previous distress can facilitate catharsis.

(c) Facilitate present tense account – to increase the cathartic effect, the patient is asked to describe the incident in the present tense as if it were happening now. Reminding the patient to remain in the present tense when describing imagery, perhaps going over it several times, which in itself can be a release, is part of this technique. Issues for a withdrawn patient may not always pertain to events and their related fears and anxieties; however, it may simply encourage the patient to express that they are in pain or feel sad or hurt. Alternatively, it may be future events and fears that are creating a state of withdrawal. Once able to reveal this, a similar three-stage approach can be used encouraging the individual to describe broadly, then literally and in the present tense, their perceptions and feelings of events in order to release catharsis.

Scanning is an effective technique that can follow the latter three-stage approach. Once clients have stated the problem troubling them, they can be invited to scan along the possible chain of incidents that has led to their present state of difficulty or distress. For instance, they may be asked to describe the chain of events that has led to their admission. They can start with the earliest incident and move forward or start with the most recent and move back. This approach can release feelings and act as a release for the present state of withdrawal or passivity.

'Slips of the tongue' can be useful clues as to how a patient is feeling and may warrant attention in encouraging greater expression, for example 'I noticed you just said..., can you tell me more?'.

Validation – at times, in fact, by and large, clients need to feel valued. Their withdrawal or state of silence may be an indication that they feel it is not okay to express themselves or if they do, you may think badly of them. Tell patients that you value them, when appropriate, and show an interest in what is happening to them. Feeling valued can encourage greater honesty and facilitates the following technique.

Giving permission – this involves allowing somebody to open up and express emotion. Nurses often appear to be very busy individuals who are constantly pressured for time. Allowing time for patients in a set aside, unhurried way and explaining that it is okay to talk, to cry or to be angry, can be an effective release, provided the nurse is prepared to be supportive and available for a period of time once the patient has opened up.

Quick asides – sometimes thoughts and feelings come up sporadically and are referred to by Heron (1990) as a quick aside. Some patients may in the course of a general conversation, skim over something that is worrying them and then quickly move on to another subject. It may be something that seems a little outside the mainstream of what they are saying. Quick asides can be focused upon if spotted, and pursued. This can be a fruitful

Table 4.2 Examples of difficult behaviours and suggested strategies

Problem	Difficult behaviour	Category of intervention to employ (Heron)	Strategies
Aggression	• Passivity • Confrontation	• Cathartic • Supportive • Confrontational (if necessary)	• Exploration of the problem – basic communication skills • Identify and address frustration • Aggression management strategies (see Chapter 5)

Fear and anxiety	• Withdrawal
	• Confrontation
		• Support
		• Information
		• Catharsis
			• Encourage expression
			• Give accurate information in clear terms
			• Use of basic communication skills
			  Active listening
			  Open questions
			  Use of touch
			  Empathy
			• Encourage catharsis
			• Support

Poor motivation	• Withdrawal • Confrontation	• Prescription • Catalytic • Support • Information	• Prescribe initially and take the lead • Promote increasing participation • Short-term goals (brief therapy) • Reward progress however small

Difficulty sleeping	• Withdrawal
	• Confrontation
		• Prescription
		• Catharsis
		• Information
		• Supportive
			• Exposure concerns
			• Prescribe possible interventions
			  Guided imagery
			  Hot baths
			  Reduced caffeine
			  Sleep hygiene factors (environment)
			  Discourage cat naps

Table 4.2 *continued*

Problem	Difficult behaviour	Category of intervention to employ (Heron)	Strategies
Attention-needing • Demanding • Interfering • Over-involved • Sexually inappropriate	• Challenge • Confrontational	• Supportive • Support • Confrontation • Prescription	Paradoxical intervention (p. 122) • Explore issues underlying behaviour • Communication must be clear • Consistent care by identified team members • Set clear boundaries/limits • Establish set times with patient • Ensure privacy without jeopardizing safety • Avoid 1:1 in over-involvement • Reward appropriate behaviour • Referral if appropriate (i.e. mental health problems)

experience, although persistence may be necessary. They have much to do with validation and giving permission and it may be that a patient is testing the water to see if it is okay to talk about a particular issue or problem. Encouragement may be needed to get patients to elaborate further.

Catching the thought – this is partially related to a quick aside but more specifically relates to the non-verbal behaviour of a patient as opposed to his verbal content. For instance, a client may be talking to you when it appears apparent that a sudden thought has come to him. A pensive expression may be seen on his face. We can all be side-tracked by our thoughts as they inter-mittently enter our consciousness. A pensive cue could be an ideal opportunity for you to ask a patient to verbalize his thoughts. For instance, the simple question 'what are you thinking about?', could suffice and encourage greater exploration.

Repetition with amplification – although a patient may seem to be withdrawn and uncommunicative, the act of withdrawal may be an indicator of discomfort, distress or displeasure. Careful observation of human behaviour has much to reveal and anxiety can reveal itself in various verbal and non-verbal ways. Distress-charged words and phrases, for instance, may be an indication of distress. It may not be the content of a phrase that alerts you to some area of pain or anxiety but the emotional charge and the way that somebody emphasizes a particular word or phrase. If emotionally charged words are recognized, invite the patient to repeat that word or phrase perhaps several times and, if appropriate, a little louder each time. Repetition such as this may release some underlying distress. Swiftness is necessary when using this skill and it may be something that takes practice and confidence to perfect. Heron (1990) warns that beginners tend to leave too big a time gap before encouraging repetition and commonly make the error of asking the patient why they said a word in such a way or tone. He argues 'why' questions are fatal, they throw the client back into a thinking rather than a feeling mode and, as such, can interrupt the momentum needed for revealing the distress in the first place.

Lyrical content – Heron (1990) advocates that when clients mention or recall a poem, piece of music or a song, you can invite them to bring it along or recite it. Music or verse may be chosen by a practitioner to facilitate catharsis. Alternatively memories or pictures can be useful cathartic aids. For example, in grief or denial about loss, personal or physical, talking with the use of visual aids as prompts can encourage expression.

For the more experienced nurse or one who wishes to practise and develop more advanced cathartic skills, psychodrama and monodrama are two possible options. Monodrama involves one person (often the patient) acting out a situation, while psychodrama usually involves two or more individuals, including the nurse. When exploring a specific event with a patient such as being told you have cancer, losing a loved one or disappointment about progress and so forth, the patient can be invited to re-enact the incident and replay it to you privately as a piece of living theatre. This may sound strange at first, but it can be very effective if handled confidently. The patient imagines he or she is in a previous scene and speaks about it as if it is happening now. The patient can also be asked to express in this re-enactment what was left unsaid, unanswered, suppressed or denied at the time. With monodrama the client is invited to play both sides of an internal conflict using two chairs which he physically switches between. The patient sits in one chair when he is speaking for somebody else or expressing another point of view and another chair when speaking as himself or verbalizing his own side. As such he may actually be playing two different people or two conflicting factors within himself that are causing distress. For example, whether to have an operation or not. In the one chair he could express views as to why he should have the operation and in the other chair, why he should not. Both approaches will not suit all patients, all situations or all nurses. They are there for selection only if it is deemed appropriate and there exists some potential for effectiveness. One cannot predict outcomes in human relationships. Both nurse and patient must feel comfortable with these approaches and full explanations are necessary. Patients must be given the choice to say yes or no to participation and to be allowed to stop at any time if they wish.

Diversional tactics may be useful in the initial stages when attempting to create a bond with very passive or withdrawn patients. Patients are often withdrawn because they are afraid of what they think, feel due to certain events or what is happening to them. Initiating discussion with a patient about what is troubling them can be quite confrontational and warrants time, sensitivity and the development of trust. One step at a time is important while watching and listening for cues. For instance, does the patient 'look' ready to open up, does she or he want to, or does she or he look tense in response to your interactions with her? In the initial phase of making contact, not only with the patient but also with new subject matter or concerns, sensitivity is paramount. To build rapport, a relaxed atmosphere can help and is less threatening. Disclosure will often only occur when and if a patient feels ready to disclose or feels that it is safe to do so. Health care professionals sometimes make the mistake of assuming that the nurse–patient relationship guarantees a level of access and familiarity. While cooperation is vital, it cannot be assumed that we have an intrinsic right to certain information or compliance from patients.

Dexter and Wash (1995) recognize some of the concerns raised by nurses when dealing with anxious patients. This is also true, to some extent, when caring for withdrawn patients who commonly harbour underlying concerns, which may affect the nurse. Table 4.3 outlines some nurse-related anxieties.

Many practitioners experience doubts and anxieties, we are all human after all. A nurse's uniform does not protect the individual from stress. While it is an important part of the nurse's role to

Table 4.3 Some causes of 'nurse anxiety' during interactions with patients (adapted from Dexter and Walsh, 1995)

Personal	Environmental	Patient
Am I helping?	Have I got time?	He is becoming more
What am I doing?	Should I be doing	frustrated
Will I be able to help?	something else?	He is becoming very
Am I saying the right	What about the other	emotional
things?	patients?	What if he turns his
What shall I say next?	I must go soon	frustration towards me?
	How do I end this?	Can I cope with all this?

communicate effectively and to portray a calm exterior, it is impor-tant to accept any doubts or insecurities and learn from experi-ences, both good and bad. A positive response when working with a withdrawn or passive patient can be built upon and stored for future reference. A negative response warrants patience, personal evaluation of self and approach and the development of a new approach if necessary. Generally, patients will respond to warmth, time and an approachable practitioner. The response rate may vary but that is to some extent inevitable. Not everybody is the same.

Ending a session – it is crucial when ending a cathartic session, that the client be brought back to the reality of the 'here and now'. There is no real need to be afraid of emotion as it is largely self-limiting. However, it helps to ask patients to describe the immediate environment and to affirm positive directions for the present by looking forward to the next few days. If the individual has been replaying experiences from the distant past, it is useful to return them to the present time gradually by chronological progression at intervals of 5 or 10 years as appropriate.

For instance: You are now 20, think of what you did for your 21st birthday? Now you are 30, where were you working then? It is September 21st 1999 and you are 36, describe to me what you see in the room.

Nurses often deny their ability to cope with intense emotion and adverse reactions, yet given the nature of nursing and often without any real forethought or preparation, such responses are dealt with on a regular basis and, by and large, coped with satis-factorily (Burnard and Morrison, 1991).

Catalytic interventions

Catalytic interventions are commonly at the core of present day models of nursing. Catalysts enable others to learn, develop and use a range of skills including teaching, showing, supporting, encouraging, confidence building, giving and suggesting, to name but a few. Nurses using catalytic interventions aim to promote patient independence or at least partial independence. Catalytic skills are generous skills that seek to facilitate self-directed living, enabling people to become more responsible for who and what they are, to gain greater control of their lives and, as such, change, grow and adapt to new experiences and situations (Heron, 1990).

Illness and disability present tremendous changes to patients, their families and loved ones. The challenge for nursing is to facilitate a return to well-being often via a change in lifestyle. Catalytic interventions are relatively new to nursing and nurses have, historically, been taught to be 'do-ers' as opposed to 'facilitators'. Hence a well-established tendency towards and reliance upon authoritative interventions in the past such as prescription and telling patients what to do has been reported (Burnard and Morrison, 1991). Given the nature of a patient's distress and neediness, the necessity for nurses to do will always remain an important and integral part of the nurse's role. However, there is increasing recognition of the value of facilitative skills and interventions. This is particularly useful in the care of withdrawn patients when interaction is often reduced and there exists a tendency to avoid as opposed to involve the individual. This is partially because it is easier and requires far less time and effort, partially because we may feel this is what the patient wants us to do or may be due to fear and uncertainty about how to help. It is important to avoid mistakenly doing too much for patients when this is not necessary or reducing contact or levels of interaction with passive patients. 'Difficult patients' are often labelled as such because they feel difficult to communicate with. Avoidance of these patients is a common strategy employed to reduce our own anxiety (Smith and Hart, 1994).

Catalytic interventions may help foster relationships with 'difficult patients' and include the following strategies:

Exploring maps – a large and crucial part of being a good 'enabler' is to find out what a patient's needs are in the context of his or her experience, perceptions and lifestyle. This is a key objective in health psychology (Ogden, 1998). Obviously in order to do this we need to spend time with patients and, if a patient is withdrawn, it is useful to have targets and tasks on which to focus.

Heron (1990) suggests important issues to explore in order to utilize catalytic interventions successfully are the following, which have been adapted to suit the health care setting and involve a schedule of set questions:

(i) Ascertain the patient's purpose or focus. What is the patient working towards? In other words, what motivates the individual? Is it power, profit, pleasure, family, work, health, enlightenment, activity, respect or a mixture of values and goals? We need to know and understand from the patient's perspective, the benefits they attribute to better health (Brearley, 1990).

(ii) Ascertain lifestyle. Find out how a patient is striving towards and reaching his or her goals. Is he or she active, inactive, happy, dissatisfied, successful or unsuccessful in this process? Is he or she achieving or achieving only in part?

(iii) What resources does the patient have available? What support does he or she have in managing a chosen lifestyle in terms of social and physical resources: for example, family, income, work, personal potential and so forth. How do these things enhance his or her lifestyle?

(iv) Plan and targets. How is the patient pacing themselves and over what time scale? Does he or she work best to short-term goals or are long-term returns preferred?

(v) Constraints. Is there anything that is stopping or hindering the ability to meet or set goals? Obviously the present experience of illness will have a large impact upon progress, but examination of this experience of ill health in relation to the past, present and future, is also important. What, how and when might the patient need to use identified resources to overcome identified constraints. Dainow and Bailey (1992) highlight the impact of constraining forces when examining the value of a strategy called 'forcefield analysis'.

Frameworks for exploration make invaluable nursing assessment tools and can be utilized, adapted and/or integrated into any nursing model, informal or formal. Many present existing nursing models incorporate elements of patient perspective and participation (Aggleton and Chalmers, 1986). Nonetheless, the need continues for nurses in every speciality and context to embrace more fully such approaches. Heron (1990) argues exploring these issues is like building a map and incorporates a series of steps. Having identified the five areas to explore in creating a patient's map, then you have to set about making one. These five areas could indeed be the foundation or the core for building new or developing existing nursing models. This is an approach advocated by Wright (1990).

Making a patient map – a map is a representation of reality, of what is happening, of where we are. Maps are formal and visible representations and can take whatever form you and the patient want them to (Wright, 1990). It does not matter what the map looks like so long as it diagrammatically represents the patient's perceptions of the illness experience. A map might involve a straightforward list of relevant details under each of the five headings identified in the form of a table (see example 1) or via any of the alternative examples offered.

Example 1

Purpose	Lifestyle	Resources	Plan	Constraints

Example 2

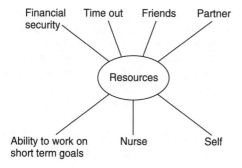

Figure 4.6 You may, using a large piece of A4 paper, use this open format and brain-storm details around it in highlighted words or phrases

Example 3

The simple use of five blank A4 sheets of paper with a heading at the top of each page may be your chosen approach. For example, the word 'purpose' is written at the top of one page, 'lifestyle' at the top of the second and so forth. Ideas can then be brain-stormed with your patient or alternatively, an explanation can be given to the patient about what to do, allowing him or her the freedom to jot down his or her own thoughts. Key points can then be discussed and negotiated at a later stage when you can add your own thoughts and input any relevant knowledge.

Naturally, this will take some time and considerable effort, particularly when a patient is withdrawn and may need more input from you initially, with suggestions and examples. Basic communication skills, as earlier identified by Egan (1998) and Nelson-Jones (1992) are a crucial part of this process. The actual format of the map is largely irrelevant. What is important is that these issues are explored and that there is a useful tool to both work from and focus upon.

Problem-specific maps – having made a broad and initial overview of the patient's individual situation, further maps of a similar nature can be produced to focus upon individual issues and problems: for instance a physical difficulty, a relationship problem, financial dilemmas and so forth.

Map making can be what you want it to be and is a process of breaking down and breaking down again elements of the individual's needs in diagrammatic, visual formats. The patient needs to be involved in the process and the map(s) must be pertinent to his or her problems perceived but with input from the health care practitioner. This means that on the whole, rather than using rigid, existing formats that may not cover or sufficiently explore certain aspects or needs for the individual, a loose framework is used that allows greater freedom to identify patient avenues, categories or issues. This may be more helpful when working with withdrawn patients as opposed to the closed yes/no responses more commonly required by many existing assessment formats. While withdrawn patients might prefer the latter, this approach does not encourage expression of their needs. Communication, generally, is opened up as opposed to closed down using open formats.

How to 'enable' passive patients to learn and develop for themselves – the necessary skills

Withdrawn and passive patients, in particular, commonly experience problems in expressing themselves or may not even see the need to do so. Some patients are happy not to be involved in their own care or progress at all (Luker and Waterworth, 1990). Sensitivity is imperative if these patients are to feel valued and safe in their ability to share what and how they feel and need. The creation of a relaxed and caring atmosphere can facilitate a forum for involvement and sharing and can be achieved by employing the following specific skills.

Free attention

This is part and parcel of the active listening skills discussed in Chapter 2. It is about encouraging expression by the giving of abundant free attention in a structured or more informal way. Free attention involves eye contact, attentive posture, facial expression and the appropriate use of touch. On busy wards, nursing attention often lies elsewhere and, with the pressures of nursing, to focus attention genuinely for a given period of time can be difficult but beneficial if achieved. For instance, think of a situation when you have stopped talking because you felt you were not being listened to. If our 'listener' looks away, looks beyond, does not respond, frequently looks at his or her watch or out of the window, this can be both distractive and unproductive.

Empathetic divining

This requires greater accurate listening with some degree of fine tuning. This skill involves exploring the whole picture of what a patient is saying, including obvious and more subtle, hidden clues that one might recognize in relation to what is said, what is not said, what might be implied, body language or through intuition. It can be compared to Egan's (1998) description of 'advanced empathy'. Empathetic divining is always expressed as a statement and never as a question. It usually opens with a phrase such as, 'It sounds to me as though you...'.

This technique can also be used when a patient is not speaking but you detect facial and other bodily cues. The response then may be, 'It looks/seems as though you...'. Heron (1990) says this approach involves reading between the lines, sometimes using what you know of the client. It can also be used in a confrontational manner to bring to the attention of the patient some aspect about himself he may be defensively trying to ignore. This can be a useful skill with withdrawn patients once you have worked with them for a period of time and there exists a degree of understanding and rapport. It is, however, a technique that does require some practice in order to deliver it sensitively. If delivered poorly, you may lose a patient's trust, which may be hard to regain.

Empathetic divining is not dissimilar to the concept of water divining, which may be the reason for its name. If you compare it to somebody using a divining instrument to search out water, the objective is the same only, in this instance, information is sought.

Heron (1990) breaks down the skill of empathetic divining into two distinct stages:

* Paraphrasing – in this stage the nurse responds to and rephrases something the patient has said. Rather than repeating it, the content of the message is fed back to the patient in your own words. This shows the patient not only that you are listening

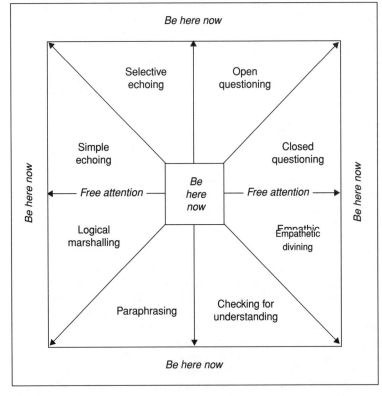

Figure 4.7 The catalytic tool-kit (Heron, 1990). Reprinted by permission of Sage Publications Ltd.

accurately, but also that, if you are not, the patient can tell you so. It may also demonstrate understanding and allows you to check your own interpretation of matters against his or hers.

- Logical marshalling – this second stage allows the nurse to determine the exact content of what the client has said, summarize it, relate parts, and indicate directions. When patients hear you do this, it can sometimes enable them to see alternative perspectives.

The use of effective non-verbal cues

Heron (1990) suggests there are five basic kinds of non-verbal cues:

- Pensive cues – patients may exhibit brief reflective expressions that reveal a variety of inner thought(s). These may go undetected. One way of addressing a patient if a pensive cue is identified might be to ask 'what are you thinking?'. Issues can then be more directly explored.
- Wanting to speak cues – body movements such as eye contact and facial expression may indicate that the patient is on the verge of saying something. The use of silence at this point and encouragement with verbal prompts such as, 'You were going to say?', may facilitate patient disclosure.
- Feeling cues – Heron suggests that these cues are an integral part of the latter two cues but may also exist alone. Patients may show signs of shock, surprise, anger, anxiety, impatience, irritation and so forth via their body language. These feelings, if recognized, can be acknowledged and brought out into the open. An example might be, 'how are you feeling at the moment?'. The use of open questions about feelings can also be effective.
- Cathartic cues – non-verbal signs may reveal that a patient is about to discharge emotion in some way. This may be evident by the display of clenched fists, tear-filled eyes or trembling. In such instances the nurse can be specific in his or her address. For example, 'Your eyes are filling up with tears, you must be feeling very hurt'. By acknowledging this, the patient becomes a little nearer to identification, ownership, acceptance and then release of feelings (Heron, 1990).
- Alienation cues – body language, posture or the removal of self from somewhere or someone, may indicate that the patient feels distant or in a state of withdrawal. Confrontation about this behaviour can be verbalized. For example, 'It looks as

though...' or 'You seem far away and distant'. Statements such as these may be followed with open questions such as, 'How are you feeling at the moment?'. A sensitive and supportive approach is necessary and the use of touch as appropriate. It is evident that there is sufficient potential to recognize unspoken feelings through a variety of non-verbal cues. This may be especially important when caring for withdrawn patients.

Following, consulting, proposing or leading

Having initiated, encouraged and facilitated successful patient expression, one of the greatest concerns that nurses express is, where do we go from here and can I cope? It is reservations such as these that often prevent the nurse from delving into the private world of the withdrawn patient and result in the employment of avoidance strategies employed to minimize interaction such as task-based communication only (Smith and Hart, 1994). This, in turn, may perpetuate a withdrawn patient state. However, once having made sufficient progress, there are four options that can be pursued.

- Once the patient has begun to disclose and explore problems, the nurse may follow where the patient goes. This is especially useful initially.
- Consult with patients about where they might like to go next. You may refer to a previous map for guidance.
- Propose a new avenue to explore and seek patient approval. For instance, 'What about...?'.
- Without recommended consultation or proposal, the nurse may lead into new territory by simply asking an open question.

Following exploration, goal setting and the development of action plans are commonly necessary.

Short-term goal setting and action strategies

Contracting therapy is a simplistic and increasingly familiar nursing approach. It is a mutual agreement between nurse and patient whereby concerns, needs and roles are made clear and explicit. It helps to establish a bond in such a way that the actions of one demand the cooperation of another according to the terms of the contract (Dexter and Wash, 1995). If patient and nurse perceptions do not match in either the understanding of the patients' viewpoint of what is happening to them and what their needs are or how to address those needs, then progress can be greatly impaired if not delayed.

Contingency contracting as described by Cameron and Gregor (1987) is 'a specific negotiated agreement that provides for the delivery of positive consequence or reinforces contingent upon desirable behaviour'. In other words, positive outcomes result from nurse and patient cooperation. These positive outcomes may be a mixture of short-term goals, such as the patient is able to get up out of bed postoperatively or have her first drink after surgery, or longer-term goals such as going home for a weekend or ultimately being discharged from hospital.

Contingency contracting is originally derived from the Health Belief Model and is based upon the concept of positive reinforcement. The contract provides rewards for behaviours that are agreed upon between nurse and patient (Becker and Rosenstock, 1987). Agreement is not an instantaneous process but involves a series of steps. To assist the nurse with this vital process Cameron and Gregor (1987) advocate the use of the following guidelines:

- First, elicit and try to understand the patient's concerns about his or her problem(s) and how he or she hopes to be helped. The patient's perspective is ascertained using the basic skills of therapeutic communication identified thus far. Patient and nurse perspective about patients' needs is often mismatched and so exploration of and listening to the patients' concerns and viewpoints is paramount.
- Give the patient as much information as possible in accessible language about their illness/problem and possible treatments. This information must be accurate, relevant and sensitively provided and can enhance feelings of control by the patient.
- Negotiate, above all else. This is both crucial and necessary and involves:
  (i)   Sharing information about perspectives with each other.
  (ii) The provision of a clear treatment plan with a clear rationale linked specifically to the individual patient's problems and lifestyle. For instance, if medication is required four times a day then gear the timing of such medication to the patient's daily routine (within reason). This too can promote greater self-control and compliance (Cameron and Gregor 1987).
  (iii) Assist in the decision making process which may at times involve compromise. Often a consensus can be revealed with time and patience.
  (iv) Set simple, specific, measurable goals based upon your identification of the patient's perspective and their priorities. Use language the patient understands when setting

out a plan and identify mutually agreed upon rewards to encourage progress.
(v) Both nurse and patient sign the contract to give it some credibility and a set of dates to review the contract are identified.
- Implement the contract.
- Ensure the contract is evaluated at the pre-arranged dates set and re-negotiate as necessary.

Below is an example of the type of format you may wish to use; however, contracting need not be so formal and can be conducted on an informal, verbally negotiated basis. Formal contracts may also be devised or adapted to suit the needs of your clients and the context in which you work. You may have one specific contract for every patient need identified or just one contract identifying several needs with plans for negotiated intervention.

Example of a contingency contract

Problem affecting healthy status:
Patient is unable to sleep and only achieves 2–3 hours sleep per night due to constant worrying.

Goal:
To sleep 4–6 hours per night.

Perceived barriers:
(This includes what might stop the patient from achieving set goals)
- Keeps thinking about problem areas at night.
- Feels fully awake at bedtime.
- Drinks coffee late at night
- Thinks 'I am not going to sleep tonight'.

Perceived benefits:
(Identify with the patient what might be the rewards of achieving goals)
- Will feel better in the morning.
- Will be more effective at work.
- Will be able to switch off at night.
- Will feel more like socializing in the evenings.

Negotiate action plan:
(Take into consideration all of the above)
- Stop drinking caffeine after 6pm in the evening.
- Will try to stay awake every night (paradoxical intervention).

- Have a hot bath at 11pm.
- Drink a large mug of hot milk.
- Write things down that are worrying me before I go to bed and plan to deal with them the next day.
- See therapist three times a week to explore problem areas in life.
- Get up at same time every day (7.30am).
- Go to the gym four times a week.

Review dates:

Weekly

Signatures:

Nurse...

Patient..

Self-contracting

Janz *et al.* (1984) advocate the use of 'self-contracts' whereby patients administer their own rewards and goals while the nurse is available for support and advice or input as needed. This is true facilitation of self-care and may not be suitable for all patients. However, it can be highly effective for some patients or patients with specific problems, i.e. the self-administration of medication. Withdrawn and passive patients often particularly exhibit poor cooperation and, at times, compliance. This is especially true when their needs are long term (Cameron and Gregor, 1987). As such, contingency contracting may be very effective if taken a step at a time. It is not about doing for or telling patients what to do, but instead about encouraging their gradual input in their own care. A large part of this process involves giving information, which will be discussed more fully in the next category.

Brief therapy

Brief therapy, in many respects, goes hand in hand with contingency contracting and has much to do with emphasizing the benefits of working mostly with short-term as opposed to long-term goals. The idea underpinning such an approach is that patients need to feel they are making progress, however small and however slow that progress might be. In addition, a set of achievable, short-term objectives are established that will eventually lead on to the achievement of long-term goals. Goals that are

---

Key concepts of brief therapy (Brimblecombe, 1995)

- Short-term goals are focused upon as opposed to long-term.
- Goals are realistically achievable or at least within a patient's grasp or potential at any moment in time.
- Goals may be necessary on a day-to-day basis or even hour-to-hour in some cases, as opposed to set weekly or monthly.
- Long-term goals are often not successfully achieved due to loss of interest, unrealistic targets, lack of patient involvement in setting objectives pertinent to them and lengthy time periods.
- It is crucial that patients are involved in setting short-term goals with the nurse. Contingency contracting can help this process.
- Achievement of short, sharp targets can bring their own rewards including satisfaction, increased hope and self-esteem and motivation.

---

overwhelming or take too long to achieve can lead to loss of interest or poor patient motivation.

Brimblecombe (1995) likens brief therapy to the nursing process which outlines similar key concepts.

Principles to guide a brief therapy interview (Iveson, 1994)

- Describe tasks in ways that clients will both understand and believe possible. To do this you must understand your client and her perspective.
- Focus upon patients' strengths and past achievements as opposed to failures. Some understanding of what has not worked previously is also necessary and can be a valuable learning process.
- Find out what the client wants for the future.

Questions that can assist this process include the following:

- What exactly is the problem?
- How is it a problem and to whom? e.g. nurse or patient?
- What has been tried before and what happened?
- How could things be different?
- How can I and others help to achieve goals?
- Have objectives been achieved? Set regular short-term reviews (Adapted from Brimblecombe 1995)

In order to achieve the above, Iveson (1994) argues that there are three principles that must guide your interview (page 102).

Informative interventions

Informative interventions naturally play a part in enabling clients to take more control over their own care and experience of ill health through greater participation.

Having established both the patient's and nurse's perspective, problem areas and their priority, informative interventions seek to give patients new knowledge and information that is directly related to those needs, in terms that can be understood. Heron (1990) argues there is quite a skill to this process. If overdone, it can overwhelm the individual, alienate him or her and restrict motivation, while if underdone, patients are left in the dark, uninformed and feeling ignorant. This has often been a criticism of health care, particularly in relation to encouraging passivity as opposed to preventing it.

Heron (1990) does acknowledge that when choosing to give information there are two basic issues which must be considered:

- How much information to give, both in terms of quality and quantity. It must be pitched at the right level, using the right terminology and in stages.
- Whether to give it at all. This issue may relate to ethical dilemmas, patient self-discovery or specific team and organizational guidelines. The issues of whether to give information or not is not straightforward and there are often no direct answers, only views. The giving of information, largely, revolves around timing. There may be good and bad times to give certain aspects of information. This requires sensitivity, the ability to empathize accurately and often a degree of intuition. Practitioners also need to take into consideration the wishes and needs of others such as relatives and partners as part of this process.

There are various practical approaches to giving information. They largely relate to the process of adult education (Knowles, 1986). This has far more to do with talking with individuals who are entitled to have a say, as opposed to talking at them, which has been problematic in the past. Some practitioners still find this transition a difficult one to make.

A variety of information giving strategies exist and include the following:

1. **Practitioner rationale.** This involves explaining to the patient what you have to do and why you have to do it. This approach

is far more effective if the patient is given this information prior to the intervention being performed and their approval or consent sought. In many cases this is overlooked. It is recognized, however, that realistically this is not always possible. It is often assumed that practitioners have the power to do whatever they want to with patients once they cross the hospital threshold. Historically, this seems to have resulted in passive and withdrawn patients. This is no longer deemed to be a desirable approach and today greater dialogue is commonly encouraged and seen in practice. For instance, consider the following options:

'Is it okay if I take your temperature because...'

as opposed to

'I am going to take your temperature' or even 'open your mouth please'.

2. **Physical diagnosis and prognosis.** Rather than solely focusing upon intervention, Heron (1990) advocates that the practitioner explains to the patient what appears to be the problem and the implications of any findings. Problem identification is based upon a range of sources and includes the patient's account and perception of events, results, observations, and discussions with others. Prognosis and the accurate sharing of information in this emotive area involves a whole range of factors that need to be debated in light of the overall picture of the patient's experience.

3. **Personal interpretations.** Practitioners use their knowledge, experience and intuition to determine each situation, give meaning to patients' behaviour and to attribute some explanation about what has been or is the problem. Understanding what is happening to you or why you feel a certain way is half the battle. However, caution must be taken when making judgements, assumptions or when expressing views that are unsupported by sufficient information and knowledge of both the problem and the individual. Interpretation may also be used as a confrontational intervention to bring a patients' behaviour to his or her attention.

4. **Psychosocial prediction.** In this instance, views can be given to patients about the possible or likely future outcome of their present problem. Understanding treatment choices in light of future outcomes (speculated or otherwise), may be uncomfortable or confrontational but may be an essential part of health promotion and the resulting lifestyle change necessary

to permit progress (Ogden, 1998). Interpretations must be offered sensitively and are often subjective. However, it is often useful to support such ideas with examples and evidence, where possible, to enhance credibility. Withdrawn and passive patients may lack trust or may deny that there is a problem and, as a result, experience difficulties facing up to their problems in the future. The involvement of patients who have had similar problems and who have worked through them successfully can be a valid approach, provided there is discussion about this and consent from the patient.

5. **Educational and growth assessment.** Assessment of the individual is an integral part of any nursing role. Nurses inform patients of what they need regarding knowledge, skills and development. This can be a purely informative approach but may be prescriptive if handled poorly. Passive and withdrawn patients may warrant prescription initially as discussed in previous sections. Information giving should facilitate choice and be an important part of enabling 'difficult clients' to express themselves more positively and take greater control.

6. **Presenting relevant information.** It is vital that when imparting information it is presented in a way that is well received and understood. It needs to be relevant to individual patient context and needs at any given time. Therefore, it must involve the following principles:

   (i) Attunement. Recognizing the individual's present ability to take on board new information. This warrants good observation of how the patient is responding to interventions and requires building upon positive responses. If confusion, poor understanding or a lack of willingness presents, this must be addressed.

   (ii) Overview. This involves the provision of a brief account of what you are going to cover, the main areas and relevance to the patient.

   (iii) Emphasize the basics. It is crucial not to include too much information at any one time and to use only a small number of key points which stand out if the information given is especially technical.

   (iv) Illumination. This means bringing to life information by illustrating main points with examples that are relevant to the listener. The use of visual aids to make your point, highlighted either visually or verbally, can be vital especially with difficult concepts. Repetition may be necessary. Visual aids may include handouts (with non-jargonated key points), demonstration videos, diagrams (not too cluttered), charts, models or leaflets. The use of colour is often effective. Visual aids are best used with supportive discussion (Reece and Walker, 1997).

(v) Command of manner. This involves the effective use of verbal information. Rate of speech should be natural but not too fast; tone should vary and volume should be adequate. The use of intermittent pauses and silence will allow opportunity for digestion of material, time for questions and any necessary clarification.

(vi) Recapitulation. Before ending your conversation or presentation, summarize the main points again to assist the memory and ability of the patient to recall relevant information.

(vii) Check for comprehension. Check for understanding by asking patients to feed back the main points of the information given or any areas they are not sure of. This should be done sensitively and not in such a way that clients feel they are being assessed or tested. People are more likely to learn when they are relaxed and often do not learn when they feel afraid, intimidated or preoccupied.

7. **Feedback.** This is a valuable tool for promoting progress once information has been given. Feedback may be given about accuracy of progress and may warrant further instruction or encouragement. When administered in a supportive way, feedback can be enlightening and beneficial and reinforce the nurse's interest in the patient.

8. **Referrals.** This strategy is used to encourage patients to access information themselves. It is a form of self-directed learning. The practitioner provides a range of information which can be more meaningful. This may include recommending books, people to contact, meetings, courses and places to visit. Each is selected to provide relevant information, support or an appropriate service to suit the patient's needs. Nolan and Nolan (1997) argue that self-direction can be problematic if patients feel they have been left to their own devices and as such, support must be evident for it to be effective.

9. **Homework**. Homework can be a productive approach which can facilitate or consolidate learning. Patients may be given a task to try out, something to read, a list, or a diary to keep. Level of involvement will determine the sort of homework identified. The follow-up of homework tasks is crucial.

10. **Experiential modelling.** Role modelling can be a powerful teaching tool. For instance, the nurse who is trying to help a

patient give up smoking can provide the necessary relevant information, but might be more successful if he or she were a non-smoker or had given up smoking him self. Credibility is, therefore, enhanced. Role modelling also encapsulates the basic elements of effective demonstration. A technique must first be mastered before it can be shown to somebody else successfully. Heron (1990) identified demonstration as a prescriptive strategy and as such, it has already been dealt with above in the prescriptive category.

11. **Self-disclosure.** Revealing information about self can be a fruitful experience for both nurse and patient, particularly if the information being shared is concise and pertinent. There is always the risk of giving too much information about self and the decision to do so may be spontaneous. However, if facilitated effectively with the intention of providing support rather than receiving it, then self-disclosure has much to offer as a technique. Decisions about self-disclosure are a very personal issue and will often be based upon knowledge of a patient, relationship with them, moment in time and skills such as advanced empathy. There is no absolute rule about the use of self-disclosure as an informative intervention. Some nurses will disclose, while others will not. The time, the place and the person involved is a personal choice and cannot be forced.

12. **Brain-storming.** A valuable and underestimated technique, brain-storming can be a useful way of exploring with patients possible options, interventions or aspects of care. It can facilitate decision making particularly when brain-storming specific issues. One well-known framework that relies upon brain-storming skills and can encourage patients to determine their own strengths and weaknesses and potential health promoting strategies is force-field analysis.

Forcefield analysis

This is an analytical tool developed by Lewin (1969) to enable individuals to examine forces in the decision making process that are both hindering and helping them in this process (Figure 4.8).

Dainow and Bailey (1992) argue that problems belong to clients, it therefore follows that solutions must belong to them also.

An example of how forcefield analysis works.

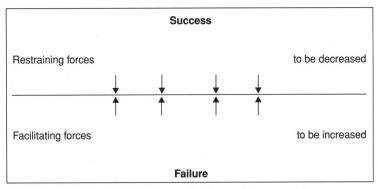

Figure 4.8 Forcefield analysis (Dainow and Bailey, 1992). Copyright John Wiley & Sons Limited. Reproduced with permission.

Needed course of action   –   To give up smoking
Possible restraining forces –   Don't want to put on weight
                                Have a stressful job
                                All friends and family smoke
                                Withdrawal symptoms
Possible facilitating forces –   Father died of lung cancer
                                Family want to give up too
                                Suffers with asthma
                                Costs too much money
                                Doesn't like smell on clothes
                                Can't smoke at work

By examining personal information with patients, facilitating forces can be used to motivate, while restraining forces can be dealt with separately, explored for accuracy and addressed in terms of action.

Above all, while information giving can be a very general domain and is often standardized for convenience, individual needs must not be forgotten. Information is more effective when personalized and applied to the individual's specific difficulty, their level of knowledge, ability, motivation and specific lifestyle. In summary, information and the way it is given to patients is crucial (Ogden, 1998). It can be a vital component when engaging patients and promoting cooperation or greater cooperation. By and large, information is transferred using oral and written strategies, some of which have been outlined, and demonstration which also features commonly in the health care setting.

Whatever the format, Ley (1989) advocates that information when given must be:

- Clear and unambiguous
- Specific
- Repeated
- Simplified
- Followed up with additional meetings or information.

In addition it is important to check for understanding when giving information and never to assume that if patients do not ask questions then they have no concerns. Encourage questions as much as possible, summarize well and ask patients to recap what you have told them. In this way you can check for understanding and weaknesses. Problems with compliance can, in particular, be addressed using the flow chart shown in Figure 4.9 overleaf.

In summary, catalytic and informative interventions are commonly interrelated and work well in a combined approach to encourage both patient participation and progress. This is particularly true when caring for patients who struggle to express themselves and withdraw as a result.

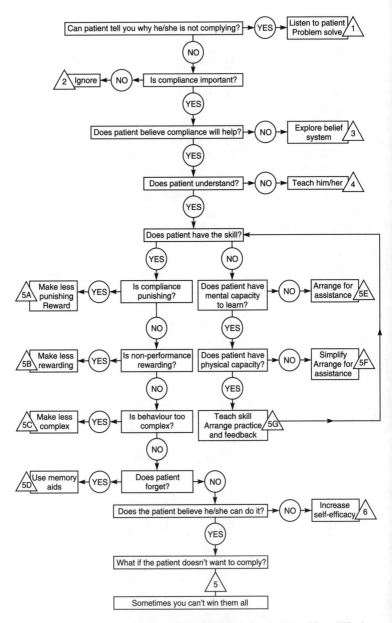

Figure 4.9 Example of a plan of possible strategies for dealing with a difficult patient (from Loring, 1992). Reprinted by permission of Sage Publications Inc.

Chapter 5

Defensive behaviours – confrontation and challenging behaviour

Issues and strategies for intervention when caring for the challenging and confrontational patient

Challenging and confrontational behaviours, in many respects, can be one and the same thing. The term challenging behaviour is used to emphasize the fact that the issue is a challenge to those who provide services (Slevin, 1995). Key elements of this broad term involve behaviours that are unacceptable to the community, physical threat or violence, disruptive or disturbed and antisocial behaviour (Clifton *et al.*, 1993). Displays such as these are possibly the most difficult to deal with in terms of the level of threat they pose to the practitioner. As such they often incorporate the very types of behaviour that instinctively make it difficult for the practitioner to respond in a therapeutic manner. Often when individuals perceive they are under personal threat or attack, the options available in response appear limited and involve defensive actions such as fighting back or flight. Flight can include denial that there is a problem or avoidance of the difficult client and his or her behaviour. It is not uncommon that the allocation of certain patients to care for each day may precipitate a sinking feeling or thoughts of 'Oh no'. A reactive response may be, in this instance, to detach self, withhold warmth or limit any communications (Smith and Hart, 1994). This in itself can lead to further confrontation and/or challenging behaviours from the patients involved.

Spotlight on Research No. 4

An exploration of nurses' responses to patient anger (Smith and Hart, 1994)

Caring for angry and difficult patients can be a threatening experience. According to Duldt (1982), nurses have a 50–50 chance of encountering angry expressions from other health care workers and patients during the course of a working week. Due to its powerful nature, expressed and unexpressed anger can be very upsetting to both the angry person and the recipient. Responses to anger appear to be based upon unique individual characteristics such as past experience, level of frustration, perceived threat, self-confidence and the presence of other emotions.

Background

Managing angry situations involves making choices about the best course of action based upon ability. For most nurses, encountering angry patients tends to cause emotional arousal, which interferes with cognitive ability to process a patient's angry message and to respond in a professional manner.

Methodology

Design   A qualitative research design was used via a grounded theory approach to explore female nurses' reactions and feelings as recipients of patient anger. The ultimate purpose was to generate a theory which describes, explains or predicts this behaviour in a nursing context.

Subjects   Nine female registered nurses from two hospitals in south western Nova Scotia formed the overall sample.

Method   Data were collected by interview using an open-ended question format and later analysed to form tentative codes and categories. The participants were asked about their experiences with anger, both in the nursing and personal context.

Findings

The findings suggest that when threat to self is high, nurses manage anger situations by disconnecting from the angry patient. Low or controllable threats were generally managed by connecting with the angry patient.

Disconnecting describes the lack of ability to associate mentally, emotionally and physically with an angry patient. Disconnecting tends to be presented for two reasons: it was the most common initial reaction of a patient's anger; and all nurses in the study revealed having gone through a similar pattern at some point in their nursing career previously. Thus, the predominant movement on the continuum seemed to be from disconnecting to connecting.

Common responses to anger perceived as threatening were:

- Personalizing angry messages
- Lacking understanding about what the patient was feeling
- Losing or fear of losing emotional control.

Emotional arousal experienced in the latter category ranged from feeling shocked, feeling attacked, feeling blame, feeling angry, feeling powerless, hiding anger to showing anger.

Disconnecting strategies to block these feelings included:

- Shielding, such as keeping cool or being defensive
- Taking time out
- Transferring blame to the patient, workplace or nursing profession generally.

When preparing to reconnect to the patient, nurses often sought peer support, rehearsed their new approach and response and tried to smooth things out for the patient. In order to then connect successfully, nurses commonly reported that one needs to:

- Non-personalize anger
- Try to understand the patient's situation holistically
- Take charge of personal angry feelings.

continued

Conclusion

The findings of this study suggest that anger and responses are multidimensional and complex. Meaning given to a patient's anger is influential; however, both connecting and disconnecting nurses tend to view the expression of patient anger negatively. In comparing how nurses managed anger in different contexts, a trend was noted. In the personal context, sitting down and talking about the issue leading to anger was seen as very important. However, talking about the incident with an angry patient was often avoided in a professional context. This study indicates that nurses often do not know how to respond in a manner which upholds their perceptions of the expectations of the nursing profession; therefore, disconnecting and smoothing things over were the predominant responses.

Based upon
Smith, M. E. and Hart, G. (1994) Nurses' responses to patient anger: from connecting to disconnecting. *Journal of Advanced Nursing*, **20**, 643–651.

Miller (1990) identifies a strand of difficult behaviour that is manipulative. This appears somewhat harsh and suggests an undercurrent of judgement. Once patients are labelled in such a way, motives underlying any interaction are viewed as hostile or underhand. Dexter and Wash (1995) refer to patients who 'orchestrate' as a preferred term and suggest that they are those who:

- Have an inability to love or recognize love, warmth or friendship when it is offered.
- Have an inability to make thoughtful decisions that are independent and free.
- Have an underlying insecurity which breeds mistrust and anxiety.
- Have feelings of inadequacy.
- Have overwhelming frustration that life is not fair or that people do not care.

Whatever the underlying cause, often patients such as these need understanding, time and assistance in fulfilling their needs. In contrast, however, they often receive avoidance from nursing staff as demonstrated in previous research (Smith and Hart, 1994).

In addition to those challenging patients outlined, Lorig (1992) suggests further problematic individuals. For instance:

- The talkers – those who take all the limelight.
- The antagonistic or belligerent participants – those who are power hungry and like control.
- The 'yes buts' – those who always have an answer or who rebuff your solutions.
- Special problem people – these are patients who exhibit very individual needs and problems of their own.

Whatever the presenting behaviour, Griffin (1997) argues the LIFE model of effective communication should be a standard approach.

L – Listen actively and feedback any interpretation of patient behaviour.

I – Use 'I' statements. Do not blame the person for how they are, but tell them how you feel by using 'I feel...', instead of saying 'You make me feel...'

F – Freedom. People should be allowed the freedom to *own* their problems and practitioners do not always have the answer.

E – Everyone's a winner. Strive to negotiate 'win–win' situations where everyone's a winner in terms of outcome achieved.

While patients will inevitably continue to present with behaviours perceived to be premeditated and attention driven, practitioners must strive to look beyond this behaviour and examine with the patient not only what they are saying and doing, but also what they are not saying and doing. In other words, ask the question 'what underpins the behaviour?'. This is not an easy task and inevitably situations will arise when patients cannot, will not or do not want to communicate or cooperate.

People come in all shapes and sizes and sadly there exists a minority of individuals who appear unlikeable (Stockwell, 1984). However, on the whole, human nature is good and the majority of patients have a story to tell, a cross to bear, or something that is upsetting them when they present as being 'difficult'. This does not mean that when confronted or challenged in an unacceptable way, particularly if under attack, that practitioners must accept this willingly as part of the job. New skills can be developed and applied to difficult behaviour and situations.

While the remaining two categories of intervention advocated by Heron (1990), confrontation and support, are examined in this chapter, nurses have the freedom to use combinations of the range of skills and interventions identified throughout this book. Previous strategies are equally as effective as part of a developing repertoire and should not be seen in isolation. Heron's (1990) work is not intended to be viewed as a hierarchy with any one category being more important than another. The key is to develop an ability to mix and match the range of approaches described, depending upon client situation and response. However, for the facilitation of presentation and to avoid repetition, when discussing types of client behaviour, categories have been focused upon separately and highlighted for their specific benefits in addressing specific problems.

The following categories will be examined in detail in this chapter and related interventions outlined:

Confrontative $\Big\}$ Interventions
Supportive

Heron's (1990) work, as with preceding sections, has been adapted and expanded upon to take into consideration a range of approaches. The categories, although appearing exhaustive in their definition, have tremendous scope for addition and update in terms of corresponding strategies.

Confrontational interventions

Confrontation, both from patients and as a therapeutic technique, is reported to be one of the most difficult elements to deal with in health care (Burnard and Morrison, 1991). Confrontation often releases a whole host of thoughts and emotions which are commonly based upon past experiences. Being confrontational can equally be an emotional and awkward experience. It seems to be particularly problematic because of the feelings of anxiety it generates, often pertaining to a fear of the unknown. Nonetheless, confrontational interventions can be utilized as a positive approach to care if dealt with sensitively and underpinned by a wish to enlighten patients in a supportive fashion.

The most important aspects to consider when seeking to use confrontational interventions are the following:

* Timing
* Is there a need for confrontation?
* Depth of confrontation used (Heron, 1990).

A crucial question to ask is 'when is it okay to confront a patient in terms of its therapeutic value?'.

Heron (1990) argues practitioners need to obtain a *warrant* to confront a patient. This involves seeking professional permission to use confrontation. In health care, it is generally accepted that there are a range of behaviours that are deemed acceptable and that are tolerated given the nature of the job. Most practitioners, however, possess a boundary that once crossed by patients, warrants some form of confrontation.

Heron (1990) suggests knowing when to confront a client directly, or otherwise, is based on presumptions. We presume, on the whole, that we are allowed to confront each and every patient. Obviously this is not the case and confrontation is filled with complexities. For instance, when using confrontation one may experience a whole range of responses from patients. This is true of the practitioner also who may exhibit numerous responses when confronted themselves. This very much depends upon whom, what, how, where or when confrontation takes place. These aspects warrant consideration and confrontation is a skill that cannot be taken lightly nor used defensively.

Example
Consider the following example of an inexperienced student nurse who uses confrontation inappropriately to the detriment of self, the patient and the therapeutic relationship.

While working on a mental health unit, a patient who returned to the ward one day in a very drunken state was confronted by a nurse. On confrontation, the patient became very verbally abusive. It is never wise to confront patients under the influence of alcohol or drugs, due to their disinhibited state, nor anyone who is in a 'heightened state of arousal' (Royal College of Psychiatrists, 1998). This is where timing becomes important. In this particular instance, while the incident passed, the relationship between the nurse and patient never recovered from this untherapeutic encounter.

This student nurse was, in fact, myself and I found it to be a very hard lesson to learn.

Conditions for effective confrontation, including timing, are an important part of the overall process. The following five conditions are a useful guide:

1. First, confrontation must be accurate and based on knowledge about the individual. Confrontation based upon incorrect information can irreparably damage a nurse–patient relationship.

2. Secondly, it should only be used when the patient is in a position to be able to do something about it. For instance, for them to make changes to their behaviour.
3. Thirdly, timing must be right and accurate knowledge about a patient and their possible response can be helpful. Be aware of the surroundings in which confrontation will take place, for safety reasons, the patient's state of mind and your motivation for the confrontation. For instance, when very upset, it is difficult to confront effectively, sensitively or objectively. There is little point in using confrontation when angry as often it is an immediate and defensive response. A useful tip is to take a couple of deep breaths and walk away for a while to calm down, if necessary, before acting or reacting. Griffin (1997) refers to this as 'calm down therapy' and patients who are encouraged to use it may also find it useful.
4. Fourthly, the depth and level of the confrontation as advocated by Heron (1990) warrants consideration. There may be several issues at various levels that need to be discussed. It is more productive to deal with one issue at a time, increasing the depth of confrontation gradually as the relationship and trust develops.
5. Finally, and above all, confrontation must always be done, at least in intention, sensitively. It should not be or seen to be a callous or personal attack, although some degree of defensiveness is almost always inevitable. An atmosphere of caring is best promoted with ongoing observation of how the patient is coping during confrontation.

Clobbering and pussyfooting around

When developing the skill of confrontation there is indeed a fine balance between 'pussyfooting around' and 'clobbering' the individual in the form of an inconsiderate or defensive attack (Heron, 1990). It is naturally difficult to confront and as a result individuals tend either to under- or overcompensate in their approach. To use confrontation effectively, the following interventions are recommended. These techniques are most effective when working with patients who are difficult and who challenge health care professionals without any implication of physical assault. This does not mean to say that confrontation is not threatening or does not induce fear and/or anxiety but that actual bodily injury is not imminent.

Each intervention is built into the following recommended framework:

1. Identify the agenda (the problem area) and raise it as an issue with the patient. In other words, verbalize to them that there is a problem and state what it is, e.g. 'Mary, I need to talk to you about the other day'.
2. Next explain in greater detail and more concrete terms what the problem is but in a sensitive manner. A balance is needed between pussyfooting around the subject and clobbering the individual (Heron, 1990) as mentioned above. A good example might be, 'you seem to be having difficulty following the programme we discussed, particularly adhering to your diet', or 'I noticed in your food diary that you have not been keeping to the plan we agreed. I wonder if there is any way I can help?'. As such you give a clear account of the behaviour or attitude causing difficulty and give supporting evidence, where possible, to clarify what you mean.
3. Then explain to the individual why you think this is relevant, particularly concerning their progress and care. Hence, you have explained what the problem is and why you have brought it up. 'I am concerned that maybe you don't understand your treatment and that your health is not improving as it should be.'
4. Give the patient space to react to what you have said. It may come as a bit of a shock to some patients that you have confronted them and they may need time to digest the information. Initially, responses to confrontation tend to be defensive, however, if this is anticipated, over-reaction is less likely. Allow emotional response to unfold and dissipate. Be ready for a variety of responses in the first instance, but be firm, confident and avoid getting drawn into arguments. The use of basic therapeutic communication skills identified in Chapter 2 will facilitate progress.
5. Follow through and do not give up or give in because acceptance or the response was not what you expected or hoped for. Once the behaviour has been addressed, work through it supportively and help the patient consider how he or she might deal with things more productively. This may take several discussions and involve the provision of space or distance for a short time. Above all, be receptive to the needs and responses of patients and adjust your input accordingly. 'There is a time for further consciousness raising and a time for leaving well alone' (Heron, 1990).

Having established a set framework for intervention for challenging behaviour or to deal with confrontation, suggested strategies that may facilitate the therapeutic process are also encouraged:

- *Direct questioning* – This involves asking outright questions about what the patient is avoiding, denying, doing or not doing or concealing. For example, 'when did you last stick to your diet?'. This is largely an 'up front' approach and should be used selectively.
- *The door in the face technique* – This is an approach advocated by Niven (1995) and involves making a substantial request followed by a small one. The idea in this instance is that it is the second request you are seeking a response to and it does not seem so difficult if a bigger, less achievable request has just been made. For example, 'will you try and be less hostile for a week', followed by, 'well at least how about for the rest of the afternoon?'.
- *The foot in the door technique* – This technique involves a softly, softly approach initially, with a more involved request being made at a later date. An example might be asking a patient to adhere to a new regime of medication for a week and then the following week asking them to take it for a year.
- *Rattle and shake* – The patient's behaviour or lack of it is challenged directly using statements that provide evidence that what the patient is doing is wrong or problematic. For example, 'You were unwell yesterday because you did not take your medication'.
- *Correcting and disagreeing* – Disbeliefs are corrected or the views of the patient disagreed with by giving factually correct information to raise the individual's awareness of the situation. This must be done in a way that neither puts the patient down nor makes them feel inadequate. This is part of the health education role of practitioners and should be addressed as necessary.
- *Changing diction* – Seek to encourage patients to own and take control of their own thoughts and behaviour by literally changing the way they phrase things. Instead of saying 'I can't do it', ask the patient to repeat the change in diction to, for example, 'I choose not to do it'. Confront patients with this change each time they revert back to the previous, more self-defeating statement.
- *From then and there to now* – For the same reason patients can be invited to switch from what they are concerned about in the past or future to what they are experiencing right now. For both this and the above techniques the nurse needs to listen accurately in order to spot these opportunities. By confronting patients about their negative thinking or obstructive behaviour, which may be underpinned with past and/or

predicted fears, one can increase a patient's positivity and resulting control over their predicament. Theories related to cognitive behavioural therapy underpin this approach (Newell, 1994).

- *Holding up a mirror* – This, a technique described earlier in cathartic interventions, can also be a useful confrontational approach. By 'mimicking' or 'parroting' an individual's behaviour or comments, one can face them with the reality of their actions. In this instance, it is important to have an established degree of rapport with a patient to feel confident with such an approach without offending. It must not be done with any malice or mocking, but be used purely to support and enlighten the individual.
- *Interrupt the record* – When a patient unwittingly begins going over old ground again, a common problem in health care, it is difficult often to facilitate progress. A useful counteractive technique is to interrupt this repetition commonly referred to as a 'long playing record' (Griffin, 1997). This can be done using diversional tactics. It may involve simply changing the topic, drawing the patient's attention to something else in the environment or by actually validating what the patient is invalidating (putting down). For example, if they argue, 'I just can't do it', you could respond, 'but you normally do it so well'. The simple use of touch can also be a valuable distraction in itself.
- *The appropriate use of disapproval* – This is facilitated using honest and open communication. The simple honesty of telling a patient when they are upsetting you can be very effective. Some patients are not aware of their behaviour or its impact. If used, this approach must be delivered sensitively.
- *Discharge feedback* – This involves allowing patients to channel their anger. This can be achieved in various ways such as ripping up pieces of paper or pounding on a pillow. The nurse–patient relationship is central to this approach and needs to be well established with provision for the necessary space and privacy. There also needs to be a strong element of trust for both parties involved. The ability to contain distress and not let the situation escalate out of control is imperative. A good knowledge of the patient and his or her common reactions is valuable; however, one must always be prepared for all eventualities. It is also important to let colleagues know where you are and what you are doing.
- *Positive attention* – This approach involves the use of self as a strong role model. Rather than becoming defensive and angry when a patient confronts or challenges you, it can be very

effective to respond in a positive and supportive way. This not only disarms the individual but also portrays a calm and accepting approach. For instance, think about a time when you have been on the phone and making a complaint. Often you get passed from pillar to post and by the time you have reached the fifth person to speak to, you may be feeling relatively angry. However, if the individual responds in a kind, apologetic and interested manner, the anger often dissipates and your frustration begins to subside.

- *Paradoxical confrontation* – In some situations it can be therapeutic to call the bluff of a client. Patients at times threaten to do things that may jeopardize their progress and possible safety. Provided this is not a life-threatening act or something that will threaten the safety of others, it may be in order to encourage them to discuss how they will go about completing their threat. In many instances, threats are made for their effect as opposed to their action; however, there is always the potential that threats may be carried out. Effective risk assessment is the key. Accurate assessment of degree of risk and damage limitation is a crucial skill necessary for this approach. Heron (1990) argues that by condoning any 'acting out', the behaviour can be paradoxically disarmed. However, he warns this intervention requires good judgement and a cool head. It also requires sound knowledge of the individual you are working with, cooperation from others and consultation with supportive colleagues.
- *Factual confrontation* – This approach is most effective when caring for patients with 'challenging problems' as opposed to 'challenging behaviour'. Accurate information-giving skills are central pertaining to condition, prognosis and future. Heron (1990) argues that to use this strategy effectively, the nurse must adhere to the following process:
  - (i)   First, give a statement to prepare the patient for the possibility of confrontation initially. For instance, 'I need to talk to you about something important'.
  - (ii) Secondly, provide a simple but informative account of the facts. This should not be lengthy as the individual at this point may only take on board limited information.
  - (iii) Next give time for the shock of confrontation to sink in and the information you have delivered. This may mean remaining silent for a while or leaving the patient for a short period. It may be useful to have someone who can support the patient (other than you) close at hand.
  - (iv) Follow through with support and time for discussion,

possible denial, and any questions the patient may have. This may be necessary straight away, later that day or at a later pre-arranged date to meet again. Ongoing evaluation of the situation will inform you as you go along. Not everybody responds to confrontation or bad news in the same way. Be sensitive and receptive to this and observe for any verbal or non-verbal cues.

(v) Finally, confrontation is a difficult thing for nurses and an anxiety provoking experience. As a result practitioners are often inclined to talk too much or too quickly. Remember it is largely the patient's distress, response and needs that are important in this instance. Endeavour to give sufficient time and space to each individual as needed.

- *Low balling* – This final strategy involves being economical with the truth, at first, in order to encourage cooperation (Niven, 1995). For instance, a patient who does not want to come into hospital because he is too busy might be told he will be able to leave at lunchtime. However, until he agrees to adhere, he may not be told that there will be further inconveniences such as the necessity to attend the ward at 8 am and to starve from the night before.

Nurses can be both the confrontee and the confronter. Whatever the situation, anxiety is inevitable and often evoked in all parties involved. While it is not usually recommended to fight fire with fire, there will be some situations when confrontation is the only approach for dealing with the situation. If this is the case, tact, sensitivity and good role modelling skills are crucial. Confrontational interventions can also be just as important and effective for withdrawn and passive patients when challenging their behaviour and as such can be adopted accordingly.

The strategies discussed in this section have, overall, been geared towards situations when the practitioner confronts either the 'difficult patient' or the individual specifically with challenging problems. The following strategies, although useful in some aspects of all nurse–patient interactions, more directly relate to the confronted health care worker and the maintenance of safety and well-being. This confrontation may take one of two forms, verbal or physical attack. Both areas have been recognized as increasingly problematic for all health care professionals (Wykes, 1994; Turnbull and Patterson, 1999; Mason and Chandley, 1999). If this aspect of health care is to be examined fully, suitably and practically, then the potential risk to nurses from challenging or confrontational patients must be addressed. Aggression and violence from patients, sadly, has escalated in recent years and may take many forms, all of which are unacceptable and destructive to the therapeutic relationship (Royal College of Psychiatrists, 1998; Duxbury, 1999a).

Dealing with aggression and violence in the health care setting

Aggression and violence in the health care setting are problems for the practitioner that warrant a very specific and careful approach. Their effects are both emotional and physical. While confrontation continues to carry risks and underlying hostility, transient or otherwise, the threat of or an actual violent act needs immediate and direct attention. The variety of approaches that have been discussed so far may indeed suffice or at least reduce the severity of an encounter, however, the maintenance of safety in some situations may become a priority and warrant further investigation.

The Health Service Advisory Committee (HSAC, 1987) has identified a common range of violent and aggressive behaviours encountered by health care professionals in one of the largest surveys to date in this area. They include:

- Major injury. This is injury that requires medical assistance for internal injuries, broken bones, sutures, unconsciousness and other injuries requiring hospitalization.
- Minor injury. This category refers to cuts and bruises requiring first aid.
- Threat with a weapon. No actual physical injury is experienced in this instance, but threats of injury or harm using an item that is or could be interpreted as a weapon are encountered.
- Verbal abuse.

The incidence of the above categories has been reported as:

- Major injury 1 in 200.
- Minor injury 11%.
- Threat with weapon 4.6%.
- Verbal abuse 17.5% (HSAC, 1987).

More recently, studies have revealed similar results and highlight the fact that minor injury and verbal abuse are the two most common and problematic forms of aggressive behaviour experienced by health practitioners (Morrison, 1993; Duxbury, 1999a). The view that these behaviours are, indeed, minor is most

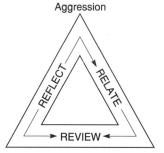

Aggression

A Nurses' Guide to Therapeutic Management

Figure 5.1 Overview of Farrell and Gray's model. Reprinted from *Aggression: A Nurse's Guide to Therapeutic Management*, 1992, by permission of the publisher Academic Press Limited, London

certainly debatable. Whatever the interpretation of what constitutes violence and aggression, and each nurse will have his or her own view of what is perceived as confrontational, challenging or threatening behaviour, the overall approach must be the same. The key message is that prevention is the better approach for both nurse and patient and for a fruitful outcome. Farrell and Gray (1992) propose the following integrated three-stage model of aggression management (Figure 5.1).

Reflect

This first stage involves the crucial preparation of nurses about the two-way process of interaction. It encompasses the potential use of self in producing both therapeutic and non-therapeutic/difficult encounters.

Relate

The second stage focuses upon the important skills of communication necessary to deal with threatening patients. It involves a combination of interpersonal skills, particularly in diffusing difficult situations and, on occasions when required, physical interventions, such as restraint.

Review

Finally, review of the experience is often overlooked, yet is a vital learning and healing experience for those involved in violent incidents. It requires the necessary post analysis of aggressive encounters and the support of and for the individuals involved.

Each stage is now explored more fully in detail below:

Stage 1 – reflecting skills and approach

Self-awareness

In order to understand patients and their individual responses, we must first be able to understand ourselves and accept our power to influence others. This includes not only how we present ourselves in the way we behave but also what we say. 'Anyone can become aggressive when feeling provoked or threatened. Often it is not clear just who is being aggressive' (Farrell and Gray, 1992).

Example 1
A patient's assertive request about her care may be interpreted as being aggressive by the nurse who is used to dealing with largely passive patients.

Example 2
A patient who is upset about something and has a valid reason for that distress, may be seen as aggressive and receive a defensive or aggressive response from the nurse. A vicious circle then ensues.

As health care workers we must constantly strive to understand each interaction, point of view and response.

In order to do this effectively one must strive to achieve the following:

- Listen to patients actively, taking in both verbal and non-verbal communication.
- Ask for clarification when and if not sure what a patient is saying or doing.
- Make time available for patients who are distressed and/or uptight.
- Provide explanations if unable to give immediate response or adequate time to patients, then make sure that an alternative time or person is available as soon as possible thereafter.
- Admit if there is a difficulty, problem, confusion or inaccuracy. This should be accompanied by an explanation (not an excuse) and an offer to remedy the situation. Nurses are only human. Patients mostly value genuine honesty.
- Try to avoid defensiveness and the urge to over-react. It can sometimes help to take four deep breaths or a couple of

seconds before responding in an emotional way, which is often our first line of defence when challenged (Griffin, 1997).

- Try to remain the 'adult' in any exchange of views, promoting an adult–adult type conversation. Confrontational encounters can often resort to parent–child type relationships (Berne, 1972). It helps if practitioners maintain open, calm and adult responses, encouraging the other person to do the same. One cannot continue to argue with someone who will not argue.
- Try not to prejudge. Get a balanced view whenever you can. The patient may well have a valid reason for being angry.
- Take on board the comments being given to you. This may be easier on reflection when the situation has settled down.
- Always accept and value the individual. If a patient's behaviour or communication is threatening or upsetting to you, feed back this information sensitively to the offender. For example 'I understand you are upset, but...' or 'I'd like to talk about this more but can we sit down because I'd feel more at ease'.
- It is useful to use terminology that comes naturally, based on the approach advocated.

When giving feedback to patients about their behaviour or progress, do so by incorporating the following points:

- End with positive feedback.
- Only comment upon behaviour observed, not on hearsay, it may be inaccurate.
- Be specific, not vague or over general, for example 'On Friday when you...'.
- Make sure feedback is given privately where there are likely to be no disruptions.
- Remember that feedback can be a shock to the individual and may upset them.
- Be prepared for a response.
- Only give feedback in the nurse–patient relationship if it is relevant to the patient's progress and well-being.
- Be sparing with feedback. Overuse can be seen as hostility.
- Give feedback caringly. If it is underpinned with anger, it is not the right time or you may not be the right person to give it.
- Allow the individual time for response and be prepared to listen to that response.
- Do not give feedback and walk away.

Be aware of potential indicators of aggression

Prevention of aggression involves accurate observation of the environment and of the behaviours of others in addition to 'self-awareness'. It is a combination of three main elements called the ABC framework:

A: antecedents – what has happened prior to the event.
B: behaviours – those which indicate anger.
C: consequences – the result of behaviour.

In order to gain a full picture of the above ABC framework, it is crucial to gain a good baseline assessment of a patient's behaviour over an identified period of time. This will incorporate anything that may have precipitated the behaviour and anything that results from it, which, in turn, may be maintaining it.

For instance, antecedents to aggressive or potentially aggressive behaviour in health care commonly include:

- Somebody upsetting a patient. This may involve difficulty with an individual, a situation or indeed several people.
- A stressful environment such as overcrowding, noise, heat, cold, lack of privacy, over lighting, monotony, restrictions and so forth. These are features often associated with ward environments. There is no shortage of criticism for hospital ward environments and the detrimental effect that they can have on health (Ogilvie, 1980).
- Internal, physical stressors such as pain, anxiety, fear, hunger and lack of sleep (Ogden, 1998).
- A lack of information and associated frustration and helplessness (Cameron and Gregor, 1987).
- Nurse-related behaviours that may cause anger in others such as defensive, aggressive, abrupt, distant, disinterested, insensitive and patronizing behaviours (Smith and Hart, 1994).
- Patients with a previous history of aggression. Those who are known to have 'short fuses' or who anger easily may be particularly prone (Royal College of Psychiatrists, 1998).
- Physiological factors that may precipitate aggression such as hypoglycaemia, post-epileptic states, head injuries, confusion or anything which may disinhibit or further disorientate a patient. Some would argue that patients with mental illness are more prone to aggression (Skodol and Karasu, 1980); the research, however, is inconclusive (Turnbull and Patterson, 1999).
- Intoxication due to drugs or alcohol (Neades, 1994; Royal College of Psychiatrists, 1998).

Table 5.1 Short-term prediction of violence (Royal College of Psychiatrists, 1998)

There is not sufficient evidence to formulate guideline statements. The following risk factors, however, are associated with violence:

Demographic or pesonal history
- A history of violence
- Youth, male gender
- Stated threat of violence
- Association with a subculture prone to violence

Clinical variables
- Alcohol or other substance misuse, irrespective of diagnosis
- Active symptoms of schizophrenia or mania, in particular if:
  - delusions or hallucinations are focused on a particular person
  - there is a specific preoccupation with violence
  - there are delusions of control, particularly with a violent theme
  - there is agitation, excitement, overt hostility or suspiciousness
- Lack of collaboration with suggested treatments
- Antisocial, explosive or impulsive personality traits

Situational factors
- Extent of social support
- Immediate availability of a weapon
- Relationship to potential victim

Behaviours that may specifically indicate increased anxiety and/or aggression in a patient include some of the following:

- A raised voice or shouting
- Verbal content indicating the same
- Clenched fists
- Clenched teeth
- Pacing up and down or around
- Banging fist or furniture
- Constant tapping of fingers
- Trembling
- Sweating
- A patient who is red in the face or very pale
- Crying
- Throwing and smashing things
- Close proximity with others
- Staring or glaring at someone
- Arguing openly
- Pointing a finger in a threatening manner
- Prolonged silence
- Swearing at others

- Verbal threats
- Sudden, forceful movements.

There will undoubtedly be an array of individual responses and ways of expressing distress or displeasure at something or someone. By the same token, there are many similarities and recognizable behaviours that can alert the practitioner to imminent aggression. Previous knowledge of a patient, in addition to good observational and listening skills, can aid prediction and, where possible, prevent escalation of a patient's anger. The old adage 'better the devil you know' can be a useful guide. However, being forearmed and forewarned does not necessarily mean that every patient should be labelled 'aggressive' or 'difficult'. This can lead to set responses and nurses can over-react to what, at times, may be situations that are simple and easy to resolve.

Equally, consequences themselves can precipitate violent encounters or maintain existing violent behaviour. For example consider the following:

- A defensive or violent response which may, in turn, further exacerbate an already fraught situation.
- Injustice (or perceived injustice) can instigate a volatile reaction.
- Impingement of liberty.
- Lack of attention or time, which may make a patient feel undervalued. Conversely, too much attention following a violent outburst may in fact encourage similar behaviour in the future.
- An inconsiderate response.
- An inappropriate response, verbal or non-verbal, such as smiling or laughing at somebody.
- Failure to keep a promise.
- Inconsistent care.
- Inexperienced staff.
- Poor staffing levels.

When needs and emotions are running high and individuals are in difficult and unfamiliar situations, the health care setting can be a minefield. It is the responsibility of the health care practitioner to be aware of his or her own behaviour and the role it plays in the behaviour of others. However, assessment of the individual and the environment on an ongoing basis is also an integral part of the process. Only then, wherever possible, can true prevention be effective.

Stage 2 – how to 'relate' to aggressive and violent patients

To communicate therapeutically with challenging or confrontational patients, Farrell and Gray (1992) suggest that there are two aspects that must be addressed. They are:

(1) Self-presentation – how we present ourselves to others when we communicate.
(2) Self-preservation – how we strive to keep ourselves safe.

It is my belief that these two key concerns are, in fact, inseparable and that one is not achievable without the other. The way the nurse presents him- or herself to patients, the things he or she says, the way he or she acts, combined, will project a lasting image both as a communicator, good or bad, and a role model. It is the skills of knowing what to say and what to do, particularly in crisis, that may be the difference between diffusing a situation and exacerbating it. This, in turn, may threaten both nurse and patient safety and well-being.

It is wrong to blame practitioners for clients' behaviour, unless malicious intent underlies the practitioner's actions, and to place responsibility for encounters entirely with the nurse involved. However, there are some valid guidelines that can be followed by professionals when needs are expressed aggressively by patients. The approach commonly advocated once prevention has failed is 'de-escalation', particularly once a situation has or is beginning to threaten to escalate out of control. Turnbull and Patterson (1999) argue that de-escalation is not just the ability to diffuse an aggressive or violent situation, 'but a set of skills that can be learnt'. The important point is that de-escalation, by definition, 'implies an approach that views an aggressive and/or violent incident as an ongoing interaction between the aggressor, the potential victim and the circumstances in which the confrontation occurs' (Siann, 1985). As such, aggression and violence can rarely, if ever, be seen in isolation.

Suggested therapeutic responses to the difficult patient who is aggressive

Endeavour to maintain an outward, calm appearance even when feeling afraid. The presentation of a relaxed role model can have a calming affect upon the aggressor and assist them in adopting a less threatening stance that is similar to yours. This is referred to as 'mirroring'. Griffin (1997) uses the term 'mood matching', which involves adjusting your level of arousal to that of the patient to promote greater trust.

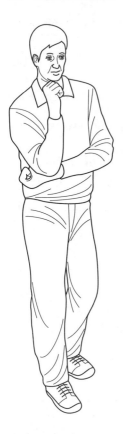

Figure 5.2 Example of recommended stance

Allow plenty of personal space for the agitated patient. This is not only less threatening but can protect the nurse from immediate injury if the patient suddenly lunges forward or throws something. To remain at a distance from patients equaling an approximate arm's length is a good yardstick.

When talking to an aggressor or potential aggressor, always adopt a side stance with feet hip distance apart, ensuring stability, and endeavour to relax your arms naturally at chest level (Figure 5.2). This means that if suddenly attacked the nurse is less likely to be pushed over and a limited amount of body surface area is exposed to injury. The facial area can also be more easily protected and there is greater freedom to use less intrusive, peripheral vision as opposed to more intimidating eye contact.

Overall, try to:

- Avoid staring at patients too much. The use of natural, intermittent eye contact is effective. It is good to make a connection with the eyes but can be threatening to give too much.
- Adopt and maintain a soft tone in your voice. Refer to the patient by name where possible and show interest in finding out what the problem is.
- Try to encourage the individual to sit down. If you both sit down this can diffuse the physical presence of a situation and make violence more difficult.
- Ensure that you are always aware of your surroundings, particularly in unfamiliar environments. This is especially important for community workers. Try to remain near to doorways whereby there is a clear escape route if necessary.
- If approaching somebody alone when violence is anticipated, always let others know where you are and when and how to get hold of you. Preferably, where possible, it is wise to take somebody with you in these situations.
- Be aware of the positions of telephones and alarms if available.
- If it is anticipated that you will not be well received by a patient or may be in some way antagonistic, the use of a different member of staff to liaise with the patient can be beneficial. Recognizing when to step down is not a weakness but indeed a strength.
- Try to appear confident by not over-reacting, particularly to verbal abuse, and show concern for the patient's distress.
- Try not to take abuse personally as this will help you to keep things in perspective and avoid defensive responses.
- If a weapon or hostage situation materializes, the police must be involved immediately. Do not tackle such situations alone and unprotected. Always send for help if you feel the situation is getting out of control.
- Try to keep other patients and bystanders out of harm's way.
- Talk to yourself in quiet internal dialogue and remind yourself 'you are going to be okay'. This will help you to feel more in control along with regular deep breaths.
- Try to encourage a 'talking through' of the problem. This is a particularly useful approach when used on an ongoing basis to avoid confrontation in the first place or to prevent further confrontation.
- Issue and make use of personal alarms, bleeps and mobile phones to vulnerable staff.
- When communicating with confrontational patients, as far as possible avoid turning your back to them. This may not only precipitate anger but may lay you wide open to sudden attack.

- Avoid the use of closed, defensive or aggressive postures such as folded arms or waving fists and fingers. Be aware of personal behaviour, bearing in mind that actions can be unconscious or inadvertent.
- Be as supportive as you can, anxiety permitting. It can be reassuring to an aggressor if you appear to care but are also in control. Remember at this point, it is they who are often out of control and really searching for answers and direction.
- Use good active listening skills. For instance, nodding, the use of open questions, phrases such as, 'I see', 'please go on' and 'I'm listening'.
- Above all, only use restraint as a last resort and if threat to the physical safety of patients or staff is imminent. Restraint must only be used in a protective sense and not as a punishment or with intent to do harm (Royal College of Psychiatrists, 1998; Mason and Chandley, 1999).
- Remove audiences where possible as they often fuel difficult situations.
- Avoid getting into an argument at all cost and focus upon 'adult-to-adult' type communication.
- Be sensitive to race, gender, age and cultural differences and/or needs.
- The use of diversional tactics can be appropriate, such as changing a sensitive topic whereby no compromise can be reached, encouraging a change of environment (a short walk) or changing activity.
- Touch can be used therapeutically in a supportive manner. However, individuals respond differently to touch and care is recommended. It can be seen as a hostile gesture or an invasion of space.
- Leave if necessary. If attacked, above all else it is your priority to get away. Shout and scream to attract attention. It is commonly believed that to shout 'fire' is a far more effective response than to shout 'help' or 'rape'.

Specific strategies pertaining to the community setting or isolated areas

Specific strategies include the following:

- Always check that you have sufficient information about a patient's history prior to a visit or consultation. This may not only prevent a difficult situation occurring, but if one does arise it can assist you in dealing with it. Try to understand how a patient operates. This includes exploring what works, what does not work, what has been tried before and so on.

- Always have an approximate schedule of where you intend to be at various times during the day and make copies available to others. You cannot be helped if it is not noticed that you are late or missing. This can be just as important in the hospital or clinic setting. Let staff know where you are.
- Call at regular intervals back to base. Make this an integral part of your day. If you are in distress, pre-arranged codes that have been identified to let others know, can be most effective. For instance, if you ring back to base and give the message, 'Can you tell Mrs Jones I am going to be late', this could alert staff that something is wrong
- Try to avoid night visits or walking alone in dimly lit areas. Carry a torch if travelling at night.
- Travel in twos if there is ever cause for concern. Again this can also apply to inpatient settings. Often, nurses go into patients' rooms alone, knowing they are going to get upset or that the encounter is going to be a difficult one.
- Always follow your intuition. If you feel afraid or something just does not feel right, your intuition about this is probably right. Make your excuses and leave (De Becker, 1997).
- Always know your destination and how to get there before you set off and avoid advertising your car as being health care related, for example through the use of 'Nurse on call' stickers. Thieves frequently target community practitioners. Uniforms can be made redundant.
- Always try to park in well-lit areas.
- Make sure you always have enough petrol and that you are covered by a reputable roadside assistance company should you break down.
- Wear clothing and footwear that you can move quickly in if need be. Again, uniforms can be obstructive. Trouser suits are useful for community workers.
- As advised by the police when travelling alone, lock your door once in the car.
- Above all, it is the practitioner's responsibility to report any concerns in relation to clients or situations. Employers have a duty of care to protect their employees (Fletcher and Buka, 1999).

In summary, Ashworth Hospital Aggression Management Team (1996) advocate that an overall approach to aggression management should be based on what they refer to as the four Cs:

- Be *confident* in your approach.
- Be *consistent* in your approach. This is particularly important among team members. If nurses are inconsistent, patients may feel confused, unsafe and may even use this inconsistency to 'manipulate' the situation. Communication between staff members, therefore, is imperative.
- Show *concern* for what the patient is trying to communicate through their anger and aggression.
- Seek *cooperation* from the client. It is much better that they become allies as opposed to enemies.

When unable to de-escalate a situation, violence or threats of violence must be dealt with promptly and positively. Increasing urgency leaves fewer options available and the choices become limited to one of four:

1. To withdraw from the situation which is largely the best option if you are in danger.
2. To protect yourself by some form of barrier if trapped or while trying to withdraw.
3. To seek assistance or
4. To employ a break-away technique or physical restraint method with the assistance of other staff if the attack persists (Ashworth Hospital Aggression Management Team, 1996).

It is not within the realms of this text to cover the last option; physical techniques such as these, which must always be a last resort, can only be effectively and safely taught as a practical and complete package. They should not be taught without appropriate instructors and supervision. Practitioners who feel they are vulnerable and open to physical assault at work should seek the relevant training. For more practical guidance in the interim, a variety of texts provide useful key points and guidelines (Farrell and Gray, 1992; Miller, 1990; Turnbull and Patterson, 1999; Mason and Chandley, 1999).

Verbal abuse in many health care settings can also be a real problem (HSAC, 1987; Morrison, 1993) and is often perceived as direct personal criticism. Indeed, this may be the case. Verbal abuse can be an indication that things may escalate out of control. A verbal display of anger or displeasure is commonly an accurate warning that warrants attention.

Griffin (1997) argues there are three useful techniques that can be employed to handle verbal attack or criticism:

1. Fogging. This is a technique whereby you agree with the truth element that may be contained within the criticism. For instance, 'You may well be right', 'You have a point'.
2. Negative assertion. This involves simply admitting that 'yes, a mistake has been made', and therefore, responsibility must be taken for this.

Both approaches can have two effective outcomes. First, literally to 'take the wind out of the aggressor's sails' and so de-escalate the situation. Secondly, to provide the acceptance of responsibility and accompanying apology, if warranted.

3. Self-disclosure. The use of self-disclosure as a preventative measure can be beneficial. If one voluntarily shares negative feelings and acceptance of them, this can be a potent tool in the prevention of imminent verbal hostility.

Techniques such as these, coupled with what is referred to as 'calm down therapy', can be a valuable, overall foundation in communication. Naturally, when faced with anger, verbal or physical, 'fight or flight mechanisms' are rapidly instigated. In order to control such responses, enabling greater rationality and less emotive retorts, 'calm down therapy' can be a simple and practical technique for personal use or to teach patients. It simply involves 'diaphragmatic breathing'.

1. Inhale to a count of four.
2. Exhale to a count of six.
3. Wait for a count of four – and begin the cycle again (Griffin, 1997).

This need not be a noticeable response, but slow deep rhythmic breathing can trigger a relaxation response when under threat.

Stage 3 – reviewing aggressive and violent incidents

Following the occurrence of an aggressive or violent incident, one area of importance that is frequently neglected, is the post crisis or post incidence phase. To be faced with or reminded of difficult situations is an unpleasant experience, but this is a vital part of aggression management. It is vital for the following three reasons:

1. We need to understand the incident and its context.
2. We need to support and reassure the individuals involved, both the victim and the aggressor.
3. We need to try to prevent a recurrence (Ashworth Hospital Aggression Management Team, 1996).

No one aspect should take priority and all three are equally important. It is not a paper exercise designed to attribute blame, but should be part of a caring package.

I talked earlier when discussing Stage 1 of reflection, about a useful ABC model. The same model applies in incident analysis but in this instance is identified by Farrell and Gray (1992) as the ABCD analysis. This involves:

A   Examination of any *antecedents*. For instance, the what, where, who, how and why of what happened prior to the incident occurring. Only by doing this can we determine if prediction can be a useful tool for the future.
B   Examination of the actual *behaviours* displayed by both the aggressor and the victim. It may be that in response to the patient's behaviour, the nurse exacerbated the situation in some way. Conversely, de-escalation techniques may have been used successfully. This is a useful learning tool.
C   Examination of the *consequences* of the patient's actions. How did staff and others respond? Did this response encourage or maintain the difficult situation? It may be that the encounter was dealt with swiftly and effectively. Feedback is crucial either to educate staff or consolidate good practice.
D   An outline of *decisions* made on the basis of the review, action plans and/or policies may need to be addressed and amended. Above all, decisions about how to support the individuals involved must be made and followed through.

There are various useful ways of conducting post incident analysis and a combination of the following three approaches can be beneficial.

The critical incident technique

The individual is encouraged to give an uninfluenced account of the event without prompts or restriction. A basic, initial open question is usually necessary, such as 'can you tell me what happened?'. This may be written or verbal and should be used shortly after the event to facilitate accurate accounts. If utilized this approach must be adopted sensitively and with initial support. Obviously, the treatment of injuries and upset must be the first priority.

Support is most beneficial usually on a one-to-one basis and in a safe and private area. This is important as both the victim and aggressor may still be feeling highly sensitive.

Naturally, if the patient remains in a very agitated state, they may warrant:

- Segregation for a short time in a quiet area with minimal stimulation.
- Time out completely away from the situation where they are able to talk and calm down. This could range from several short minutes to several hours, depending upon need and cooperation.
- Physical or chemical restraint as a last resort. It is essential that this is both supervised and appropriate (Royal College of Psychiatrists, 1998).

Incident forms

Most areas have post incident forms; however, they are often not completed or are administered poorly. This defeats the object of the exercise and may be used inappropriately to replace support. This is not satisfactory, as they must be used in conjunction with support. They are vital tools and it is imperative that evaluation takes place and is not overlooked.

Follow-up in one-to-one or group support

Once the individuals involved have had time to recover, follow-up of the incident is crucial. For many, attack of any sort can be a terrifying experience and, although people seem to be coping, they may, in fact, not be coping at all. Informal reviews may be instigated to assist the individual to regain confidence and learn from the experience or more formal referral may be necessary. The latter is important, particularly if difficulties continue and new problems emerge.

In a more constructive, supportive fashion, personal reviews (6-monthly/annually) can be effective forums for development. The provision of supervision via mentorship, provision of training and constant encouragement and recognition of strengths while working on weaknesses, can be useful learning strategies.

While prevention, management and review would be expected to be components of any aggression management package, busy lives and busy workplaces mean that overworked health care workers facing daily demands can inadvertently overlook the very basics of 'therapeutic communication'. It is both vital and necessary to make constant checks of your feelings and each situation, taking stock at regular points of how you are doing. However you choose to do this, whether it be via time set aside or incorporated into your working day, it can limit the experience and trauma of then having to deal with confrontation from 'difficult patients'. It may even one day save your life.

Supportive interventions

Supportive interventions, while both recommended and valuable when dealing with all types of difficult patients, are an integral part of caring for challenging and vulnerable individuals.

A supportive intervention is any form of therapeutic procedure in which direct help is provided. It is a form of therapy commonly offered to people experiencing some form of crisis. Difficult patients, in particular, are often battling with some form of internal conflict. Some clients may need support for long periods of time, while others will only require support short term.

Stewart (1993) suggests the aims of supportive therapy are to:

- Help a client maintain some degree of independent living.
- Restore abilities and inner resources.
- Enhance self-esteem.
- Establish realistic expectations of care.
- Prevent deterioration.
- Enable clients to function with minimum support.
- Involve others in the process of support.

Supportive interventions are advocated by Heron (1990) and affirmed for their value in the helping relationship. While they are recognized as a natural component of health care relationships (Burnard and Morrison (1991) found that nurses are most comfortable with these interventions), the literature tends to focus upon the concept of social support.

Social support has been used to represent many different concepts. The main three identified are:

1. Social integration into a relationship, for instance, the nurse and patient relationship.
2. The social network which explores the interrelationship between a variety of individuals.
3. Social support which explores the functions of the social relationship (Keeling *et al.*, 1996).

It is the third concept that tends to receive the most attention in terms of description and research. Balzer-Riley (1992) suggests that in the broadest sense of the word, support is anything that helps you to function more effectively and feel better about your ability to function. However, this notion of support tends to be vague and does not necessarily enable a helper to articulate what is needed or give the appropriate advice. A way of operationalizing support is to think of the concept as being broken down into three components:

- Cognitive
- Affective
- Physical.

Balzer-Riley (1992) refers to this as CAP. Cognitive support helps the individual to think about how and why they are doing things in certain ways. Affective support is the good feeling that accompanies open, direct communication and is often referred to as reassurance. Physical support is the concrete assistance given by an individual, the use of equipment or a change in the environment.

Within each category of support, there are a variety of interventions that can facilitate expression of that support to the individual. They are as follows:

Cognitive support
1. Offer direction to the individual, for instance give concrete advice.
2. Provide information.
3. Promote progress through inspiration and feedback about that progress.
4. Challenge the individual if you feel they are on the wrong track and offer alternative suggestions.
5. Express concern and care about each patient. This, in turn, helps them to feel that they are valued. This process is commonly called validation and may apply to health care staff.
6. Share your thoughts about the individual's situation and difficulties. Self-disclosure can enhance a feeling of support, provided it is used to make a point about the patient and not the practitioner.
7. Encourage clients to examine any positive progress and build upon it.

Affective support
1. Offer empathy and listen carefully to each patient.
2. Reassure patients' anxieties by recognizing needs and feelings. Address false beliefs.
3. Give praise for progress and enthusiasm.
4. Affirm the worth of the individual by always greeting them with 'professional warmth'.
5. Give feedback thoughtfully and tactfully.

Physical support
1) Ensure that optimum assistance is always available. This involves ensuring adequate staffing levels, facilities and an environment that promotes progress.
2) Use touch to express concern and convey warmth as deemed appropriate. Physical contact can be very supportive.
3) Do things and give things that you know will mean something to each patient.

Heron (1990) suggests that supportive interventions are simple, human and small in number. They normally relate to things that matter to the patient and so a crucial part of being supportive involves knowing and understanding your patients. Supportive interventions, in many respects, are difficult to define and can involve a combination of a variety of other interventions, as discussed thus far. To be supportive is to choose the most appropriate tools that will enable each individual to feel better, valued or more positive.

The nurse's supportive role may stretch beyond the boundaries of the nurse–patient relationship in terms of time needed and input. Strategies can focus upon the provision of additional support such as the introduction to self-help groups or the enhancement of existing supportive relationships through education and involvement (Keeling *et al.*, 1996).

Whatever the form of support offered, direct or indirect, it is crucial that the type of support needed is delivered appropriately and that it has the desired effect in relation to patient coping. Ongoing evaluation is therefore, an integral part of the process whereby support can be adapted to meet the necessary needs of both the nurse and patient in the helping relationship. This is defined by Langford *et al.* (1997) as appraisal support and supplements the variety of approaches employed to care for difficult and non-difficult clients including emotional, instrumental and informational support. Norbeck (1988) views social support as central to the caring goals of nursing and it remains a pivotal point in the facilitation of the helping relationship (Heron, 1990).

Chapter 6

An overview of the 'rules' of therapeutic communication

Throughout the context of this book, there lies a thread, a set of principles, which govern a way of thinking that can enhance communication and resulting relationships in health care. This set of principles I have called the 'rules of therapeutic communication'. While there exists a range of tools and strategies that can be employed dependent upon individual need, situation, response and preference, the 'rules' aim to govern everyday relationships in practice. They are the foundations on which to build the structure and content explored in previous chapters.

The 'rules' have guided and underpinned my view of 'therapeutic communication' and have been left to the final chapter for one of three reasons. First, having digested this material for the first time, they will make more sense and seem relatively familiar. Secondly, they can act as a useful reminder and revision of relevant points and issues. Finally, they facilitate a succinct 'bringing together' of all you have learnt, yet remain the foundation on which you may now begin a journey of growth in practice. As such, they may also be seen to be the beginning.

The rules approach, as with many helping models, if applied and shaped to the individual selectively, has much to offer the nurse–patient relationship. I have intentionally outlined, adapted and expanded upon those rules crucial to the foundations of therapeutic communication and its practical application. These rules not only have the capacity to underpin future communication for the better with 'difficult clients', but also to be a valuable preventative measure when dealing effectively with difficult situations and dilemmas.

The original 'rules' developed by Fein and Schneider (1995) in this adapted form are a useful springboard on which to develop the ability to communicate therapeutically in a caring environment. The rules have not only been selected and refashioned to suit the health care setting but have also been expanded upon to provide the practitioner with a sound framework on which to nurse effectively.

The 'rules', like any other framework, need to be practised and rehearsed. The discerning nurse or health worker will use the 'rules' not only to enhance communication in practice, but to improve his or her relationships in general. The 'rules' require a way of life, to some extent, and above all a change in thinking. Hay (1994) refers to the 'chatterbox' within us all that continuously underpins our fears, doubts, anxieties and overall negativity. The 'rules', if followed, can help us break free from negativity and promote productivity in how we think, feel and behave towards patients. This, in turn, can allow patients to do and be the same. There is nothing so powerful as a good role model other than a very bad one.

Fein and Schneider (1995) argue the rules are not about giving up all you stand for or changing self, they are about the advancement of self-respect and dignity, which once achieved can be used to bring out the best in others. For instance, have you ever noticed that when it is a bright and sunny day and you feel good, people around you seem less hostile or irritable? Conversely when you are in a bad mood, everybody else seems to be in a bad mood also. How we behave can influence the behaviour of others and the overall experience of each nurse–patient relationship, however brief, we enter into (Peel, 1995).

Having established that there exists a set of rules in therapeutic communication, they are examined below in greater detail.

Rule 1 Be an individual (a practitioner) unlike any other!

There is a need to move away from the days when we did certain things because that was the way they had always been done (Walsh and Ford, 1992). Nurses have the potential to be change agents and set precedents for good communication and practice. To strive to be a practitioner unlike any other involves close examination of the way individuals present themselves to others. Confidence and belief in self can only radiate from within. For instance, consider the nurse that patients look forward to seeing. It may be the way he or she smiles, listens actively, looks, uses touch or conveys sensitivity. Largely, it is a general ability to communicate with patients in a way that reflects the message, 'I am interested in you as an individual and want to help'.

Rule 2 Don't be too intrusive or overpowering

In other words strive to be approachable, but give patients the freedom to warm to you at their own pace. There is nothing more intimidating or threatening than somebody who constantly confronts another with the question, 'What is the matter, I know there is something wrong?'. Think of personal relationships and how they make you feel. It is a common mistake when practising communication skills to try too hard and to try to do too much too soon (Heron, 1990). Allow patients to open at a pace acceptable to them and facilitate discussion of any concerns by simply being approachable and accessible. If nurses are rarely available or visible to patients, patients may never have the opportunity to address concerns. This may mean taking time when caring or performing very basic nursing duties. Often, practitioners expect patients to disclose too readily and participate in intimate procedures without the necessary social preparation. While these situations are impossible to avoid in health care, preparation must be catered for, physically and emotionally. Strive to be patient and give frequent non-verbal and verbal cues that will encourage the development of a trusting relationship. For instance, the use of intermittent eye contact, sitting down with patients as opposed to standing over them, an occasional smile, the use of touch and various attending responses.

Helping patients, 'difficult' or otherwise, can be a timely process, yet can be worth every minute of time and energy invested.

Rule 3 Respect a patient's boundaries. Do not force intimacy too soon

This follows on from and is part and parcel of Rule 2. Intimacy is something earned, not expected, and professional intimacy is the result of patience and respect. Whether physical, emotional or social intimacy, it often develops between two people because they have a common foundation. They exhibit similarities, conscious or otherwise (Skinner and Cleese, 1995). Physical intimacy such as examination and various physical interventions becomes a way of life for many nurses and is commonly routinized. Nurses are, however, increasingly beginning to recognize the importance of the development of a degree of rapport with patients before close contact can be expected.

Rule 4 Don't tell patients what to do – negotiate

One of the biggest problems in nursing and a common barrier to fruitful nurse–patient relationships and ongoing cooperation, is the general assumption by health care workers that once a patient crosses the boundary from the community into hospital, that they become the property of those caring for them. Patients need advice, guidance, assistance and support at different times depending upon need. They may not always ask for help, particularly when feeling afraid or in distress. The nurse, therefore, needs to be astute in his or her observations and sensitive to such patients' needs. To become accustomed to telling patients what to do without consultation is not uncommon.

It is increasingly recognized in health care work that compliance and cooperation is best achieved by involving patients in their care and adopting regimens to suit their individual needs as opposed to forcing patients to change their lifestyles to suit hospital based routines (Cameron and Gregor, 1987).

A second important, underlying element to this rule relates to power and the unequal balance in the nurse–patient relationship that can exist. Patients are relatively vulnerable on admission, first due to the nature of their illness or disability and secondly by the hostile and unfamiliar environment they find themselves in. Stripped of personal clothing and belongings, patients have historically adopted a helpless role (Parsons, 1964); nurses, conversely, tend to adopt a more dominant position. This, however, is changing and nurses are increasingly encouraged to share control with patients (Ashworth *et al.*, 1992).

'Difficult patients' are commonly the product of a rigid regimen and frequently labelled when reluctant to comply (Stockwell, 1984; Miller, 1990). Not all patients wish to comply and some would rather be told what to do (Luker and Waterworth, 1990). Providing the choice not to collaborate can be seen as participation in itself and shifts the emphasis of care from control to negotiation.

Rule 5 Don't open up too quickly – the rule of self-disclosure

Schools of thought about the rules of self-disclosure vary. Examples reflecting various views include 'don't open up too quickly', 'share what you feel', 'express yourself', 'don't let your barriers down' – I've heard them all! The key to self-disclosure is to trust your instincts to some extent. If the moment feels right and the disclosure seems appropriate, then do it. The key is not to over disclose and to bear timing in mind when you might wish to share experiences or feelings.

The priority of any nursing role is to fulfil the necessary duty of care to patients (UKCC, 1992). Sources of professional support and coping strategies will vary outside the hospital environment and should be utilized appropriately. However, there will be times when the moment feels right to share a personal thought with a patient. It may be a past experience, a feeling, a view, a moment or just simply a tear. The ability to share can be a mutually valuable experience. In this way permission is given therapeutically to 'let go', and 'open up'.

For many years it has been advocated that the private thoughts and feelings of practitioners, whatever the situation, should remain private. It is possible that as a result of this approach, patients have been alienated unnecessarily. One does not expect a nurse to respond openly to every aspect of suffering encountered on a daily basis, as this would be physically and emotionally overwhelming and exhausting. However, instinctively to seize the moment and use the skill of self-disclosure, is not a professional failing but a therapeutic opportunity.

Rule 6 Be honest!

The role of honesty will always encourage a wealth of dilemmas in nursing, particularly as decisions related to patient knowledge are not always in the control of the nurse. Honesty is not always about giving accurate information, but also involves saying when you do not know, do not understand or just feel you are not in a position to comment. Honesty most definitely does not always involve saying yes to patients or telling them what they may want to hear. There are times when it will be therapeutic to the patient and your relationship with them to say no and establish a few clear boundaries. For instance, when in an unfamiliar environment or when following an unfamiliar schedule, it is reassuring to know 'the rules' sometimes and what is and is not expected or acceptable.

Difficult patients may emerge as a result of confusion or uncertainty about such things. Clear channels of communication and messages are essential (Peel, 1995). Strive to recognize when patients do not understand or need to know more. Patients will respect you for your efforts. Verbalizing what is on your mind in a sensitive and well-timed manner can be very therapeutic and not only sets the scene for honesty, but encourages honesty from patients who may respond in a reciprocal manner.

Rule 7 Devote time to each nurse–patient relationship

Relationships, be they therapeutic or otherwise, need time to develop. Clients labelled as 'difficult' are often avoided or ignored (Smith and Hart, 1994), which may compound and escalate any presenting 'difficult behaviour'. Studies reveal that in some instances there are certain 'types' of patients nurses avoid more frequently (Stockwell, 1984). This, in turn, may pave the way for difficult behaviour to be initiated in the first place.

The 'stitch in time' rule applies to communication in general. There is evidence to suggest that many of our more problematic conversations (those that may turn into battles) could be avoided by staying in more regular contact with those we interact with. Making contact with another does not have to involve frequent, long periods of intense conversation but short bursts of regular chat, support or information giving that leaves the patient feeling informed, valued and reassured.

Rule 8 Dare to connect

Susan Jeffers (1992) has written extensively on the issue of positive thinking. One of her well-known sayings is, 'there are no strangers, only friends we have never met'. There is no written law that stipulates that to nurse effectively one must remain detached, uninvolved and distant with patients, yet the befriending of clients is commonly frowned upon. Nurses by the nature of their profession must be allowed and prepared to 'dare to connect'.

Jeffers (1992) argues that connection is made easier when we approach other people with the primary purpose of making them feel better both within and about themselves. Nursing shares a similar goal, which involves connection with those who are vulnerable as opposed to disconnection and avoidance (Smith and Hart, 1994). A degree of self-awareness is an integral part of this process. It is important to examine why certain patients may make us feel uncomfortable. As a result detached nursing roles may diminish and feelings of empathy be fostered.

Difficult patients are not only those who annoy us or make us feel uncomfortable for a variety of reasons, but may also be those we fear due to the feelings of intense compassion they raise within us.

Rule 9 Admit that 'I want you to like me'

Part of the problem often when dealing with patients who themselves are distant, angry, uncooperative, aggressive or just plain 'difficult', is that we too may feel vulnerable and insecure and interpret such behaviour as a personal attack. Powell (1975) suggests 'I am afraid to tell you who I am because if I tell you who I am you may not like me and it is all that I have'. This is a good clue as to why connection between individuals can sometimes be so difficult.

In order to recognize and address barriers such as these, Jeffers (1992) argues there are two essential elements to developing effective interpersonal relationships. They are:

1. Stop trying to be perfect. This is one situation where 'giving up', so to speak, has to be the healthiest thing you can do for yourself. The ability to accept imperfection within ourselves allows greater toleration and understanding of the imperfections within others. This is not the promotion of negligence or crucial omissions, nurses are duty bound to strive to do their best for patients (UKCC, 1992), however, it does allow the process of therapeutic communication to take its course. The nurse–patient relationship is the experience of two people who sometimes make mistakes, get confused, tire, feel insecure but above all, continue to have the capacity to make a difference to the other.
2. Figure out your act and begin dropping it. This message is clearly be yourself. Genuineness lies at the heart of interpersonal communication and relates to various rules discussed so far (Rogers, 1980; Arnold and Boggs, 1995). It is a core value in therapeutic communication also and recognized as a vital element for effective relationship building and development (Egan, 1998; Sundeen *et al.*, 1994; Hargie *et al.*, 1994).

Rule 10 Make the first move

The majority of health care professionals work in environments that are familiar to them. This provides a degree of safety and an element of control. Nurses choose to be nurses, to nurse in any given speciality and, on the whole, to meet daily nursing responsibilities. Patients rarely share this luxury and have limited control over their admission to hospital, planned or otherwise.

The ward environment is filled with alien sights, sounds, smells and behaviours, which generally generate feelings of fear, anxiety and uncertainty. Given the imbalance of power, it is hardly surprising that barriers exist and bonds are difficult to establish. Nurses have a duty, therefore, to make the first move. It should not be the patient's responsibility to reduce a practitioner's disease (discomfort), yet Stockwell's work revealed the contrary. Findings showed that nurses identified popular patients as those who made 'them' feel good.

Patients often need to be given permission and encouragement to express any questions and anxieties. In some respects, nurses are the hosts of their environment, while patients are transient guests. Patients expect, therefore, to be invited to participate and welcomed in this role. This is the reality of health care and patients, while silent and seemingly unconcerned and cooperative are, in fact, harbouring private concerns. Jeffers (1992) argues it is important always to take the responsibility for making the first move and the second and the third and fourth if necessary in any relationship. It is important to be responsible for *your* level of involvement and, while the responses or reactions of others cannot be controlled, to some extent they can be influenced, particularly on initial contact. The first hello is an essential part of making a connection with a patient and establishing a working relationship for future interactions.

Rule 11 Focus on being interested

Commonly, a variety of factors can interfere with the establishment of effective relationships such as fear of rejection, failure or a lack of self-confidence. Destructive, negative self-talk can exacerbate these feelings and is referred to by Jeffers (1992) as a 'chatterbox'. This can be likened to a 'worry box', which overflows with the many numerous daily concerns individuals might harbour. Persaud (1997) describes these thoughts as ANTs, automatic negative thoughts, that commonly disrupt effective communication with others. It is important that practitioners identify these thoughts and work through them. For instance, imagine yourself standing at the bedside of a new or particularly 'difficult patient', even worse, at the door of a new or unfamiliar ward. You are facing a stranger or a room full of strangers and feeling very nervous. Internal dialogue is threatening your confidence and ability to communicate productively. It is exactly at this time that you need to address your need to be interesting and liked and work on being *interested*. In order to do this, Jeffers (1992) advocates the following steps:

1. Say 'stop' to this chatterbox. This can be achieved visually in your mind or verbally depending upon the setting or situation at the time.
2. Replace the negativity of the chatterbox with self-caring talk. These are called self-affirmations, which serve to remind us of our worth. For example, 'I am a good nurse', 'I have much to offer'. Repeat these positive statements at least 10 times in quick succession. Jeffers (1992) argues these statements do not have to be fully believed in order for them to work. The subconscious mind absorbs them and this is the most important thing.
3. Next assure yourself that no matter what response you get from others, you are a worthwhile person. Self-belief is a valuable tool which can be developed with practice, like any skill. By affirming self, the chatterbox can be silenced.
4. Finally, Jeffers (1992) suggests you are now prepared to address the individual you are interested in getting to know. Selection of which patients to interact with and which to ignore is rarely an option for practitioners; however, nursing time and level of contact can be reduced or even withheld from those we do not feel comfortable communicating with (Smith and Hart, 1994).

It is essential that when learning to self-affirm and to deal with difficult patients, mental reminders of each interaction can be helpful.

For example, 'this is a person just like me...who wants to connect...who wants to be liked...who is in pain...and who is just as nervous as I am'.

Rule 12 Engage in 'everybody training' as opposed to 'somebody training'

Often the environment and previous experiences can affect relationships (Jeffers, 1992; Cook, 1993). Jeffers (1992) suggests that from the day we are born we immediately enrol in what she calls 'somebody training'. That is, we are taught by our parents, significant others and society in general, that what we are supposed to be in this world, is *somebody*! As a result, our 'somebodiness' is dependent upon factors such as status, power, personality, looks and so forth. The problem in this perfection-seeking approach is that often we fall short of ideals and as a result, have impaired self-worth. This, in turn, can affect how we relate to others.

Nurses and patients cannot escape influences such as these, which may result in the experience of the difficult patient, difficult nurse and/or difficult encounter. Somebody training means that individual differences are overemphasized. Interestingly, 'difficult patients' are often those who are perceived to be 'different'; for instance, patients with mental health problems, those from ethnic minorities or those who generally do not 'conform' to the 'norms' of either the hospital ward or society (Stockwell, 1984).

'Everybody training', on the other hand, aims to engage, making a *connection* the priority of any interaction. 'Connection', says Jeffers (1992), 'is made easier when people are approached with the primary purpose of making them feel better about themselves'. To reduce contact with a 'difficult patient' or to avoid dialogue, valuable opportunities are missed. Nurses need to endeavour to listen to what patients are saying and attempt to understand feelings. This is referred to as empathy (Kagan and Evans, 1995). While boundaries inevitably have a place in the hospital environment, an eagerness to make connections can promote rewarding nurse–patient consultations. This approach is also based on the 'Law of Karma', that every action generates a force of energy that returns to us in like kind (Chopra, 1996). Nursing is a helping relationship, much of which is based on the will to help (Egan, 1986; Nelson-Jones, 1993).

Rule 13 Apply the 'law of least effort'

This law is referred to as one of seven spiritual laws of success proposed by Deepak Chopra (1996). It is based on the principle that the right way can be sought with least effort. Grass does not try to grow, it just grows. Fish do not try to swim, they just swim. Nurses do not usually have to instinctively try to care, they just do. Least effort is expended, argues Chopra, when actions are motivated by a caring approach.

There are three components to this law. The first component is *acceptance*. Acceptance of people, situations, circumstances and events as they occur. The moment is as it is and as such, there is little point in struggling to change things. To try and change the 'moment' only leads to distress and frustration. It is more productive to concentrate not on altering the situation, but instead on our response to it.

This leads on to the second component of the 'law of least effort', that of *responsibility*. This means not blaming individuals or circumstances for the situation, but having accepted the 'moment', taking responsibility to respond in a positive way.

Lastly, within the framework of this law, one needs to master the art of *defencelessness*. A large amount of time and energy is spent and wasted defending points of view and striving to convince, persuade and even coerce patients into adopting certain opinions and beliefs to promote well-being. This, in turn, can lead to resistance. Chopra (1996) argues when there is no point of view to defend, arguments do not develop. This approach reflects the aims of health psychology which are to promote health through involvement, communication, education and cooperation (Ogden, 1998).

Rule 14 Transform conflict into partnership

Conflict can refer to any behaviour that is perceived as aggressive or uncooperative. In the hospital environment this can involve a power struggle between nurse and patient, whereby one aims to influence the behaviour or decisions of the other using force or domination. Whoever the culprit, this is not conducive to the development of a therapeutic relationship or therapeutic communication.

Kohn (1990) argues that competition of this nature has the potential to damage relationships, promote suspicion, hostility and envy, destroy self-esteem, create anxiety through a need for approval and is time consuming and inefficient. He refers to it as an 'againsting process'. Competition may not only be the resulting behaviour of difficult patients, but also the precipitating factor from either nurse or patient that has led to a difficult situation in the first place.

Confrontational situations can be commonplace in health care (Wykes, 1994; Hadfield-Law, 1998) and may unveil a whole range of problem behaviours that the health care professional has to deal with (Hadfield-Law, 1998). Confrontation is threatening to all and often dealt with defensively using avoidance or denial (Smith and Hart, 1994). This is not the essence of therapeutic communication, yet is a common response to 'difficult patients' and obviously counterproductive. The answer, suggests Jeffers (1992), is the use of the 'partnership model' as opposed to the more commonplace 'dominant model'. The partnership model promotes compromise whereby problem(s) or dilemma(s) need to be understood from the patient's perspective. The ideals of treatment are then adapted to incorporate the individual's viewpoint. Patient participation is not a new concept in nursing (Brearley, 1990) and skills such as 'contracting' (Cameron and Gregor, 1987) are evident in practice. New strategies also promote this approach, for instance, brief therapy (Brimblecombe, 1995).

Conflict, in essence, does not have to be perceived as only negative. The potential of any conflict encountered can be transformed and viewed as an opportunity to practise the skills of negotiation. This may not be a straightforward process and involves time, patience and the effective use of empathy to establish alternative viewpoints. This is therapeutic communication and, in order to transform conflict into negotiation, new skills may be necessary (Jeffers, 1992).

1. First, long established beliefs may have to be challenged. Other points of view are valid, irrespective of background, experience or knowledge. Practitioners often have the appropriate information about options of care, but patients have the knowledge concerning their own predicament and resources. Sharing of viewpoints and knowledge is crucial.
2. Points of view are important contributions to the overall picture. This sometimes involves a change from the didactic use of the biomedical model and telling patients what to do (Wright, 1990), to alternative approaches.
3. There will always be times when disagreements arise. Patients, once given the appropriate support and information in light of their individual needs, should be left to make choices for themselves, when able (Orem, 1990). Guidance and advice is commonly required (Heron, 1990), but the nursing role is not to coerce, force or insist, even when choices made cannot be condoned (Gates, 1994). There are situations when patients' views may be overridden and these contribute to an increasing wealth of ethical dilemmas, but in the main, it is the duty of the nurse to respect the wishes of patients who are fully informed (Kenrick, 1994).
4. Stop being defensive! This is commonly a natural response when under attack and frequently creates barriers to any possible further productive communication.

5. Many patients have a valid reason for showing displeasure. Acknowledgement of this does not mean acceptance of their choice of behaviour, which may need to be addressed in a supportive fashion, but can mean giving value to the other person's ideas or perception of events. This is frequently referred to as 'validation' (Heron, 1990) and communicates a willingness to listen and negotiate, with a view to addressing problems.

6. Finally, it is a useful skill to engage in consultation with a patient as if you do not know anything about them. Preconceived ideas and knowledge can be destructive and it is not uncommon for nurses to be socialized routinely through ward 'handovers' into labelling patients as 'difficult' before they have even met them (Stockwell, 1984). For instance, 'Mrs. Jones never stops complaining. Once you go near her you'll never get away'. Or 'be careful of Sarah Smith and keep your distance, if you spend too much time with her she is likely to try to manipulate you'. Preconceived ideas have the potential to interfere with therapeutic relationships.

Allowing others to do things and express themselves, within reason and acceptable levels of safety, without judgement, encourages greater understanding and communication. These steps help practitioners to engage clients, establish fruitful connections and set the scene for mutual participation.

Rule 15 Endeavour to understand the individual

Covey (1994) suggests there are six major deposits that can be made to build up an emotional bank account of some worth. This rule, he argues, is one of the most important investments one can ever make and is the key to every other deposit. The more deposits made into both our own and others' emotional bank accounts, the more successful the relationship. To try to understand a patient's point of view and personal experience enables the practitioner to know what sort of investment to make in order to help. The greater the investment, the more productive the relationship and the more fruitful, ultimately, the account.

To understand somebody's needs, it is often necessary to try to put yourself into their shoes. This requires the skill of empathy (Egan, 1998). Whilst one of the most basic skills needed to nurse effectively, empathy is commonly one of the most neglected areas in nursing (Burnard and Morrison, 1991). This, in turn, creates a barrier to effective nursing outcomes when two different perspectives are being pursued.

Rule 16 Attend to the 'little things'

'It's the little things that count.'

'Take care of the pennies and the pounds will look after themselves.'

These are phrases familiar to most and project the same sort of message. Yet in the hectic daily concerns of a hospital ward, unit or caseload, it is the small courtesies that are often the first to go. Covey (1994) argues 'small discourtesies, unkindnesses and little forms of disrespect, make large withdrawals from the emotional bank accounts addressed earlier. In relationships, little things are, • in fact, big things'. For patients, when vulnerable, afraid and on unfamiliar territory, minor worries and irritations can inevitably become major anxieties.

When a patient is removed from surroundings and routines that are familiar, and many aspects of their day controlled from 6am to 10pm, it is hardly surprising that anxieties can predominate. The 'little things' are all important and when catered for can leave a lasting impression. Many are familiar with the friendly nurse who is liked by all. It may be you. This is the nurse that all patients ask about and tend to remember. 'When is Jane next on duty?' Why is it that some nurses are so well liked and received? Could it be something to do with their attention to detail, their sunny dispositions and their ability both to remember and take care of the 'little things'; for instance, a welcomed smile or a hand on the shoulder at the right moment. Noticing when flowers need their water changing or bringing telephone messages straight away when loved ones have phoned, can have a lasting impact. In the same way, the gentle squeeze of a hand, giving 5 minutes when a patient is upset or changing a cold cup of tea for a hot one are all examples of attending to the little things. I am talking about the nurse that stands out. The fact that such nurses stand out at all suggests there is a need to look more closely at communication skills (Champken-Woods, 1992; Faulkner, 1994). Possibly there would be fewer difficult patients if issues such as these were more commonly addressed.

Why is it that all practitioners cannot be that nurse, when all that is required is an additional minute or two in a busy routine or schedule? Set yourself an exercise and try it the next time you are with a patient. Choose a patient you do not have much to do with ordinarily or indeed someone you view as a 'difficult patient'. Next time you go to hurry past them, stop and decide to attend to the 'little details'. Give them a smile or stop to find out about their world. You will be amazed at the difference it makes both to the way they feel and the satisfaction it might give you in doing so. Attending to the little things is a mutual experience, one that can have a lasting impact and is important to most patients, even if they fail or refuse to show their instant appreciation. Appreciation may, in fact, never be forthcoming but your actions could have made a substantial difference.

Rule 17 Keep your commitments

This may sound to be common sense or something all nurses strive to achieve in their professional lives. Yet if you were to count up the amount of times in one day you had intended to do something, then failed or just plain forgotten to do so, you may be surprised at the sum. Nurses are commonly heard to say, 'I'll just be a minute'. Minutes can easily turn into hours and even longer. The golden rule when striving to keep commitments is only to aim to make promises, informal or otherwise, that can be kept. If it then becomes evident that there may be difficulty keeping to the original arrangement, honesty is important and valid reasons necessary. Sometimes, to ask for release from a promise can be effective. Such approaches are both important for less formal promises such as, 'I'll be with you in a minute', to those commitments that are central to the well-being and progress of the individual.

Covey (1994) advocates that keeping a commitment or a promise is one of the major deposits described in Rule 15. Breaking one, he says, is a major emotional withdrawal, and destructive to the nurse–patient relationship. Making promises that are important to patients (and this is a key issue, important to them and not always to you, understanding this is crucial), and then failing to deliver the goods can promote distrust. The next time a promise is made, the patient is less likely to believe it. Breaking a promise is an issue of trust. If there is limited trust in a nurse–patient relationship then the ability to help that individual effectively is affected. The therapeutic bond may be weakened and the foundations for the development of a poten-tially 'difficult client' with behaviours such as 'non-cooperation', non-compliance, and a need to make 'demands', may have been established.

Rule 18 Clarify expectations

Invariably, patients come into hospital, particularly for the first time, unsure of what to expect and unclear about what will be expected of them. Patients do have a role to play, a role that fluctuates depending upon the health care climate (DOH, 1998). However, they tend to look to the nurse for cues as to where, when and how to act. From a nursing perspective, the hospital environment is familiar and roles are often defined. As a result, nurses may overlook the new and unfamiliar experience that patients encounter when hospitalized.

Expectations are often presumed to be understood. If patients do not meet the expectations of practitioners, frequently they are labelled as difficult, although the process may not be consciously recognized. Whether dealing with professional issues or general relationship concerns, one thing is clear, that undefined expectations will lead to misunderstanding, disappointment and withdrawal of trust (Covey, 1994). Covey (1994) states 'many expectations are implicit'. They haven't been explicitly stated or announced, but people nevertheless bring them to a particular situation or relationship. 'Although these expectations have not been discussed or sometimes even recognized by the person who has them, fulfilling them makes great deposits in the relationship and violating them makes withdrawals.'

This is true in the nurse–patient relationship and therefore, it is important that with each new situation, patient or encounter, expectations are clearly established from the start. This involves considerable investment of time and effort but may save the same as the relationship develops.

Difficult patients are often the result of limited communication, which involves poor clarification of expectations or perspectives which include expectations (Hadfield-Law, 1998). Covey (1994) highlights the problems that may result and states 'when expectations are not clear and shared, people begin to become emotionally involved and simple misunderstandings become compounded, escalating into personality clashes and communication breakdowns'. A patient may not conform or comply because he or she may not adopt responsibility believing that it is the role of the patient to remain passive (Luker and Waterworth, 1990). It is only through sharing understandings of what is and what is not expected that an atmosphere of equality can be created. This is especially important as the nursing role expands and there is increasing encouragement to exchange views with clients (Morse, 1991).

Consumers of health care services need to be made aware of this shift in emphasis in order to be able to contribute more fully. Many negative situations are created by simply assuming that professional and personal expectations are self-evident and that they are clearly understood and shared by other people. This is not always the case and nursing priorities based on assumptions of what patients might be thinking and feeling do not necessarily tally with what patients see as their priorities of care.

Rule 19 Show personal integrity

People can seek to understand, remember the little things, keep their promises, clarify and fulfil expectations and still fail to build reserves of trust when inwardly at odds with themselves. Those who are bitter, always at odds with the world and critical of others, undermine trust and do not create the foundations for effective interpersonal relationships. 'One of the most important ways to manifest integrity is to be loyal to those who are not present. In doing so we build the trust of those who are present. When you defend those who are absent, you retain the trust of those who are present' (Covey, 1994). Integrity, when visible, is often respected and valued by others. For example, consider a staff meeting where one member of staff is criticizing a colleague who is absent. Who would be respected, the individual who is making the complaints about somebody behind their back or the colleague who was unable to defend him- or herself, irrespective of who was right or wrong at the time?

Working relationships, whatever the context, need to be based on mutual respect, genuineness and integrity (UKCC, 1996). When everybody is treated in the same way, there is minimal room for distrust, doubt or uncertainty. Patients, largely, will only choose to mistrust if given reason to do so or as a result of previous bad experiences. Whether communicating by word or action, professional integrity ensures that underlying intentions are based on respect. If there is a need to confront or disagree with a patient, and indeed there will be times when this is necessary as discussed in earlier sections, confrontation is not suitable in a public arena but in the privacy of a one-to-one appointment. This is one example of how integrity might manifest in practice.

Rule 20 Do not be afraid to apologize

There are many situations in nursing when an apology coupled with an adequate explanation, could avoid escalation of patient anxiety, dissatisfaction and resulting anger. There are undoubtedly numerous situations that are out of the immediate control of nurses such as busy routines, cancelled appointments, delayed or prolonged surgery lists, noisy ward areas, difficulties contacting doctors, unrealistic patients, overloaded caseloads, increasing paperwork, lengthy meetings and so forth. The list is endless. Yet what is controllable is a practitioner's ability to communicate and do so effectively. Burnard (1992) and Egan (1998) argue this is a skill that can be learnt. There is nothing more obstructive for some patients than to be left in the dark. Often patients are not approached when there is a problem because of a fear of possible confrontation or blame. In fact, any actual confrontation is often far worse if ignored or unattended to. It can take a great deal of strength of character to apologize. It may be that we feel it is not our place to apologize, particularly if the problem is not our fault. However, nurses are frequently the most immediate point of contact for patients and commonly put in positions whereby they are forced to act as negotiators or mediators. Alternatively, problems can be exacerbated if health care professionals contribute to a conspiracy of silence. 'If we don't say anything, maybe they won't notice' sort of approach. Do not be fooled, patients invariably do notice, and a lack of communication then damages the relationship.

Constant updates of information and honesty when things have gone wrong or are not going according to plan, can prevent potentially difficult situations from escalating into confrontation. 'It is one thing to make a mistake and quite another thing not to admit it. People will forgive mistakes, negligence aside, because mistakes are usually of the mind, such as mistakes of judgement. However, mistakes of the heart, ill intention, bad motives, or hiding initial mistakes is less easy to forgive (Covey, 1994). Open communication can enhance the quality of the nurse–patient relationship and promote greater patience and cooperation.

Rule 21 Practise, practise, practise the rules

Learning the rules of therapeutic communication and how to use them is not necessarily straightforward. It is not my intention to suggest that every practitioner needs to change their personality or dramatically change their approach; however, the need to think a little more about performance and adapt accordingly to enhance relationships, is evident. Nobody is perfect and everybody can make a mistake at sometime when dealing with others. This may involve failure to recognize an important cue, insufficient time to give thought and care to interactions, defensiveness or lack of self-awareness. There is always room for growth and development.

Fine tuning communication skills and getting good at the rules is like learning any skill. One gets good by practising. You may not get it right first time or every time, but do not be discouraged. Think back to when you were learning to drive or to ride a bike. There were so many things to remember and the ability to drive or ride successfully may have seemed impossible. Striving to be an effective communicator is much the same and with time, commitment and practice, the rules can eventually become an integral part of daily, therapeutic communication and relationships. It may be that you work well in some areas of the rules already but need to develop others more fully. To practise the rules on a day-to-day basis enables greater effective utilization when dealing with difficult situations or patients.

Rule 22 Do the rules – don't be put off

The need to improve communication in health care is increasingly evident (Tschudin, 1993; Burnard, 1992; Hargie *et al.*, 1994; Newell, 1994; Kagan and Evans, 1995). Many nurses have the ability, skills and knowledge for effective therapeutic relationships but, due to ongoing pressures, miss important opportunities to use these skills. A succinct reminder of the main points can be useful and if referred to regularly can facilitate their use. Difficult patients, in turn, may appear less threatening and be perceived differently as individuals with specific needs and problems.

Rule 23 Don't break the rules

This may be one of the hardest rules of all to adhere to. Sometimes when successful in an approach, complacency can develop and learning is stunted. Wrong! The rules of therapeutic communication demand ongoing effort and attention if they are to complement each nurse–patient relationship. Every new situation, patient and problem requires the same level of investment. To break the rules can be counter-therapeutic and sets the scene for the potential development of a 'difficult client'. This then requires additional time, energy and a return to the rules to endeavour to rectify any breakdown in communication.

The rules are a combination of approaches in human relationship work and are supported by a wealth of discussion and research in this area. Strive to perfect the skills identified which, in turn, will increase your confidence in using them.

Rule 24 Don't take rejection personally

Patients reject us, become angry and 'difficult' to communicate with for a variety of reasons. A natural and often immediate action when somebody appears hostile is to ignore them, become defensive, respond with hostility or to withdraw altogether (Smith and Hart, 1994). This may be particularly true when dealing with a difficult or unpopular patient (Stockwell, 1984). Patients tend to behave in a hostile or obstructive manner when they, themselves, feel threatened, upset or frustrated. Many patients experience a range of anxieties when first admitted to hospital or on their first contact with health care professionals, yet not all patients will use these feelings to alienate the nursing staff who care for them.

The context or people involved in what is happening will often mean the difference between a problem handled successfully and one handled poorly. The situation and level of anxiety will be affected by both internal and external factors. For instance, how the patient and nurse feel physically or psychologically, the nature and depth of the problem itself, past experience of dealing with difficulty and ability to manage the problem. The potential complexities of human behaviour and experience are evident and the nurse's skills and objectivity are crucial. The ability to display self-control and a sense of calm when all around seems chaotic, requires both self-discipline and the ability to empathize. It is far easier to do this when hostility is not viewed as a personal attack but the situation accepted for what it often is, a difficult one.

Rule 25 Strive to know yourself – the art of self-awareness

One of the most crucial aspects of therapeutic communication is the ability to know yourself. This means recognizing both good and bad points and working within personal limitations and strengths. There will be situations that some handle well, just as there will be certain types of patients who appear easier to relate to than others. This does not mean interactions can be selected but that an ability to admit that with which we struggle is important. Then and only then are we able to seek appropriate guidance, advice and support.

Problematic situations and patients tend to be avoided (Smith and Hart, 1994) and as a result needy patients can be alienated. However, the ability to recognize when to refer and when to withdraw is also necessary in health care. Patients, too, must recognize and take some responsibility for their actions (Department of Health, 1998) which, at times, may be entirely unreasonable, irrespective of problems, lack of resources, distress or perceived threat. A self-aware nurse who understands him- or herself can be reassuring to patients who are struggling.

Rule 26 Do not be afraid to use confrontation when appropriate

Burnard and Morrison (1991) have identified that of all the helping skills described, nurses most commonly struggle with confrontational and cathartic interventions. Catharsis means the release of emotion; therefore, it is of little surprise that nurses find these skills difficult to master. Inherent in the process of confrontation and catharsis there exists a strong fear of the unknown, particularly as both may expose the practitioner to unnecessary vulnerability or expressions of emotion from patients. Many nurses express fears that if they allow patients to unveil anger, distress, tears or deep personal material, that the result may be difficult to contain. Such fears, it seems, are largely unfounded or at least exaggerated. This is by no means true in every situation and human behaviour heralds some degree of unpredictability. However, many patients do not unrealistically expect practitioners to solve all their problems or make them whole again once they have broken down. Possibly and more realistically, support is expected and empathy during their *moment* of distress.

Most patients can, in fact, 'pull themselves together' once they have come apart and would rather do so. For instance, think back to the last time you felt you have 'gone to pieces' and cried long and hard. There is a sense of relief and calm once crying subsides, for a short time at least. Often the ability for self control is more readily available than most are given credit for. This ability may, however, vary considerably from person to person according to age, experience, disposition, situation, resources, state of well-being and moment in time. On the whole, to allow patients to express emotion is not something to be feared or frowned upon.

The use of a confrontational approach with a patient, however, is somewhat of a different matter and warrants sensitivity, particularly for another's feelings. Confrontation is a skilful and most useful art if handled well and as such has been dealt with in some detail in the previous chapter. The underlying objective must be to achieve the greatest benefit to the patient, not in coercing or bullying him or her to do as you wish, but in enlightening the individual about behaviour or needs which may be hindering the ability to progress to better health (Heron, 1990).

The direct release of emotion and the effective use of confrontation can complement approaches addressed and strengthen the nurse–patient relationship.

Rule 27 Expect to fail sometimes and be prepared to learn

Ideals and standards are an inherent part of nursing. However, no matter how hard we try, there will inevitably be times when we perceive we have failed. When this happens, disillusionment can set in and the therapeutic rules can be abandoned. There will also be times when things do not go according to plan or people react in a way that is unexpected or out of character and context. This is part and parcel of any relationship. Irrespective of this, there is much one can do to enhance communication with patients overall. To have tried and failed with good intentions is far more beneficial than never to have tried at all for fear of failing, or even worse, through disinterest.

There are many things people would have liked to have done better and maybe did not achieve (this time). Times such as these can be the most pertinent of learning experiences. Appreciate every encounter for what it is and do not be afraid to evaluate, adapt and fine tune the rules advocated to suit your personality, patients and environment. Believe in yourself, be willing to communicate and the rest will follow.

Closure of the nurse–patient relationship

It seems pertinent, that as I finish writing this book, the issue of closure should be my final few pages. The ending of a book or nurse–patient relationship can leave a lasting impression and it is partly up to the individual whether this be a good, bad or indifferent experience.

The termination phase or 'end' of a nurse–patient relationship is a crucial one and far too often under-played or completely ignored. The skills the nurse uses when closing a relationship can mean the difference between positive or limited progress and a satisfied or unsatisfied customer. It is often the unsatisfied customer who will return as what might be termed the 'distant unpopular patient'. This is the patient who keeps ringing the ward, turning up, asking for further input or writing to the hospital. This, in turn, may lead to repercussions of a more formal nature. It seems a great shame in some instances if excellent care is undervalued by inadequate termination skills, particularly when this experience is likely to be foremost in a patient's mind.

Commonly, it is long-term relationships with clients that receive greater consideration about and in preparation for the termination phase. This can be problematic, particularly with the increasing emphasis upon short-term encounters in health care. Irrespective of context or depth of the nurse–patient relationship, preparation and successful implementation of closure is vital.

Morse (1991) suggests there are, in fact, only four types of nurse–patient relationships. These, she argues, incorporate all levels and include:

- Short
- Therapeutic
- Intimate
- Over-involved.

The identification of each relationship is based upon factors including length of time involved, trust, focus of relationship, perceptions of roles and intensity of problem. These elements and their focus can be seen more clearly in Table 6.1.

The bulk of nurse–patient relationships, it is argued, take the form of a 'therapeutic relationship' (Morse, 1991). However, irrespective of length of relationship, short, medium or long term, patients need direction. This applies to closure also. The level of direction given will depend upon the relationship and needs within that relationship. Those that require only one meeting or that are for a short period of time are less likely to require the support of those that call for greater investment. Conversely, those that necessitate prolonged care and the development of what one might term a 'relationship', will undoubtedly both require and inherently have the time for greater preparatory work and warning prior to closure. Irrespective of the type of relation-

Table 6.1 Types and characteristics of nurse–patient relationships (from Morse, 1991)

Characteristics	Types of relationship			
	Clinical	*Therapeutic*	*Connected*	*Over-involved*
Time	Short/transitory	Short/average	Lengthy	Long-term
Interaction	Perfunctory/role	Professional	Intensive/close	Intensive/intimate
Patient's needs	Minor Treatment-oriented	Needs met Minor-moderate	Extensive/crisis 'Goes the extra mile'	Enormous needs
Patient's trust	Nurse's competence	Nurse's competence Tests trustworthiness	Nurse's competence and confides Consults on treatment decisions	Complete: 'puts their life in the nurse's hands'
Nurse's perspective of the patient; patient's perspective of own role	Only in patient role	First: in patient role Second: as a person	First: as a person Second: in a patient role	Only as a person
Nursing commitment	Professional commitment	Professional commitment Patient's concerns secondary	Patient's concerns primary Treatment concerns secondary	Committed to patient only as a person Treatment goals discarded

ship, closure must involve as far as possible the following basic components:

- Preparation and information.
- Support.
- Referral or discharge.

Preparation, particularly in short-term, planned encounters is largely self-evident. For example, if a patient visits a practice nurse for an immunization, he or she will largely expect one or two visits. Someone going into hospital will commonly have some idea, pre-admission, as to length of stay and what is likely to be involved. Patients are prepared for discharge from the start by the nature of the consultation and the problem/need encountered. Sometimes, intuitively, it becomes evident that there are individual patients who are going to need more warning and/or support than others. It may be, in some instances, that these are the patients quickly labelled as being 'difficult'.

Support may take many forms but, if closure of the nurse–patient relationship is to be successful, involves ensuring the patient has sufficient back-up on discharge, adequate knowledge and understanding, a degree of self-sufficiency and information. The latter may include a range of approaches, for instance, self-help groups, videos, handouts, helpline numbers and referral if necessary. Some practitioners prefer to have an 'open door' policy in their ending whereby the patient can always return or make contact if necessary. Of course, in many respects this is largely the case and given the nature of health care, while reassuring to most patients, the majority will never have to use this option. Others, however, may find it very difficult to let go and need more rigid therapeutic boundaries. It soon becomes evident who these patients are and may stem back to inadequate preparation about closure initially.

Support, in many instances, is often reduced gradually as the nurse–patient relationship develops. For example, length of time between appointments can extend from twice a week, to weekly, to fortnightly, to monthly and so on. This process, in itself, is good preparation for closure; however, it remains important to remind patients at regular intervals of the need to reduce support and why. It may be that they are making good progress, that you are working to a set contract, that there is nothing more you can offer the patient or that referral is pending.

Referral is an important part of the nurse's role and requires a combination of skills. It is also a common part of closure for many practitioners. The termination of one nurse–patient relationship can be the beginning of another practitioner–client relationship. In order to refer appropriately, the nurse must have a good understanding of the patient's needs and be able to communicate these accurately. In addition he or she must be fully aware of the appropriate services available and what they have to offer, understand the referral system for that service, know when to refer and to whom and finally, have the communication skills to facilitate referral. Some practitioners may choose not to refer because they lack the assertion skills necessary to terminate a nurse–patient relationship. This is not good practice. It is not only unfair to the patient, who may require specific expert help but is also poor use of services available.

In summary, the best approach to successful closure of the nurse–patient relationship includes good assessment of the patient's progress and needs in relation to termination, ongoing preparation for closure from day one (formal or informal), reminders at key points, discussion, negotiation and referral. A useful outline can be seen in Table 6.2.

Table 6.2 Sample dialogue for terminating a long-term relationship

The nurse says to the client:

1. 'Before we meet again I want each of us to take some time to be alone, as much time as we choose but no less than a half hour. We must plan for this time well so that we ensure that we are undisturbed and undistracted.'
2. 'Give careful thought to the place and the time of day chosen for this time alone. Plan well so that nothing deprives you of this time and that this time alone is exactly the way you want it to be. Most important, spend this time alone. I will do this, too.'
3. 'While alone let yourself reminisce about our relationship. Recall the first session we had together and review historically any moments that come clear to you. Give yourself the luxury of staying with these moments as long as you want to. Ask yourself: "What has this experience been for me? What has touched me?" Most important, think about you in this relationship and feel whatever feelings come up inside you. I will do this, too.'
4. 'Next, while you are alone, let yourself imagine and/or fantasize how you want the last session to be. Include as many details as possible. At first this may be very difficult to do. Stay with the task, nevertheless, allowing yourself to think and feel whatever comes to you. I will do this, too.'
5. 'Having done this imagining, practise this scene. So many of us have never had a satisfactory good-bye. Allow thoughts and feelings of previous partings to come to you. How were they? How do you want this one to be? You and I must say good-bye. Practise your chosen scene for our parting over and over, changing or modifying it until your image of the last session is perfect for you. I will do this, too.'

From Koehne-Kaplan, N. S., Levy, K. E. (1978) An approach for facilitating the passage through termination. *Journal of Psychiatric Nursing* **16**:11. Reprinted with permission.

The message of therapeutic communication

In conclusion, the message of 'therapeutic communication' is one as a practitioner you will either hear or choose to dismiss. It may be that you feel you know how to communicate effectively; however, when was the last time you asked for or checked upon feedback? Realistically, sometimes we communicate well and sometimes we do not. This is also true of patients and, as a result, sometimes they are, become or are perceived as being 'difficult patients'. Whatever the interpretation, they present as both a problem and a challenge for all health care workers. To ignore the needs of a 'difficult patient' will only precipitate the emergence of a 'very difficult patient'.

To care effectively for patients in distress whether withdrawn, passive, challenging or confrontational, the nurse needs to maintain a consistent and caring approach. In addition, utilization and access to a range of therapeutic skills and tools is important and to aim to be receptive to the individual needs of each patient and their individual reactions.

The rules and underlying philosophy are the foundations on which to build, adapt, explore and review encounters with difficult patients. To recognize difficult encounters with patients as part of a two-way process and to constantly strive to do the best that you can for every patient, is a theme I hope I have successfully portrayed. If by writing this book I can make a difference to one nurse, patient or interaction enabling a practitioner to feel 'I made a difference to that patient', then I am satisfied that I have contributed in some way to the process of greater effective communication in practice.

References

Aggleton, P. and Chalmers, H. (1986) *Nursing Models and the Nursing Process.* London: Macmillan Education Ltd.

Argyle, M. (1990) *The Psychology Of Interpersonal Behaviour*, 4th edn. London: Penguin Books.

Arnold, E. and Boggs, K. (1995) *Interpersonal Relationships: Professional Communication Skills For Nurses.* London: WB Saunders Company.

Ashworth Hospital Aggression Management Team (1996) *Practical Aspects of Managing Violence – Modules 1 and 2, an Ashworth Learning Pack.* London: Epsilon Production Network.

Ashworth, P. D., Lungmate, M. A. and Morrison, P. (1992) Patient participation: it's meaning and significance in the context of caring. *Journal of Advanced Nursing,* **17**, 1430–1439.

Audit Commission (1991) *A Short Cut To Better Services. Day Surgery In England and Wales.* London: HMSO.

Balzer-Riley, J. W. (1992) *Communications in Nursing.* 3rd edn. London: Mosby.

Becker, M.H. and Rosenstock, I.M. (1987) Comparing social learning theory and the health belief model. In: W.B. Ward (Ed) *Advances in Health Education and Promotion.* Pp 245–249. Greenwich, CT: JAI Press.

Berne, E. (1972) *The Games People Play.* London: Penguin.

Blake, R. and Morton, J. (1972) *The Diagnosis and Development Matrix.* Houston: Scientific Methods.

Brearley, S. (1990) *Patient Participation: The Literature.* London: Royal College of Nursing/Scutari Press.

Brimblecombe, N. (1995) Clinical reports. The use of brief therapy as part of the nursing care plan. *Nursing Times,* **91**(35), 34–35.

Brown, A. and Duxbury, J. (1997) Day surgery – Communicating and interviewing skills. *British Journal Of Theatre Nursing* **7**(4), 10–15.

Burnard, P. (1989) *Counselling Skills For Health Care Professionals.* London: Chapman and Hall.

Burnard, P. (1992) *Communicate.* London: Edward Arnold.

Burnard, P. and Morrison, P. (1991) *Caring and Communicating.* London: Macmillan Press Ltd.

Cameron, C. (1996) Patient compliance: recognition of factors involved and suggestions for promoting compliance with therapeutic regimes. *Journal Of Advanced Nursing,* **24**, 244–250.

Cameron, K. and Gregor, F. (1987) Chronic illness and compliance. *Journal Of Advanced Nursing,* **12**, 671–676.

Cava, R. (1996) *Dealing With Difficult People.* London: Piatkus Publishers Ltd.

Champken-Woods, A. (1992) Communicate – A theatre art. *British Journal Of Theatre Nursing,* May, 10–12.

Chopra, D. (1996) *The Seven Spiritual Laws Of Success.* London: Bantham Press.
Clifton, M., Brown, J. and Naylor, V. (1993) Learning disabilities, challenging behaviour and mental illness. *ENB Research Highlights.* London: ENB
Cook, M. (1993) *Levels Of Personality.* London: Cassell.
Covey, S. (1994) *The Seven Habits Of Highly Effective People.* London: Simon and Schuster Ltd.
Dainow, S. and Bailey, C. (1992) *Developing Skills With People.* London: John Wiley & Sons.
Davis, H. and Fallowfield, L. (1994) *Counselling and Communication In Health Care.* Chichester: John Wiley.
De Becker, G. (1997) *The Gift Of Fear: Survival Signals That Protect Us From Violence.* London: Bloomsbury Publishing Plc.
Department of Health (1983) *Mental Health Act.* London: DOH.
Department of Health (1991) *The Patient's Charter.* London: HMSO.
Department of Health (1998) *The New NHS Charter: A Different Approach.* Leeds: NHS Executive.
DeVito, J. A. (1986) *The Interpersonal Communication Book,* 4th edn. Cambridge: Harper and Row Publishers.
Dexter, G. and Wash, M. (1995) *Psychiatric Nursing Skills: A Patient-Centred Approach,* 2nd edn. London: Chapman and Hall.
Dillon, J. T. (1990) *The Practice Of Questioning.* London: Routledge.
Duxbury, J. (1999a) An exploratory account of registered nurses' experiences of patient aggression in both mental health and general nursing settings. *Journal of Psychiatric and Mental Health Nursing,* 6(2), 107–114.
Duxbury, J. (1999b) Medical Emergency Admissions: Literature Review. Liverpool: Haccru, University Of Liverpool.
Duxbury, J. and Brown, A. (1997) Day Surgery – Communicating and interviewing skills. *British Journal of Theatre Nursing,* 7(4), 10–15.
Egan, G. (1998) *The Skilled Helper,* 6th edn. London: Brooks/Cole.
Ellis, R. B., Gates, R. J. and Kenworthy, N. (1995) *Interpersonal Communication In Nursing.* London: Churchill Livingstone.
Farrell, G. A. and Gray, C. (1992) *Aggression: A Nurses' Guide To Therapeutic Management.* London: Scutari Press.
Faulkner, A. (1994) *Teaching Interactive Skills In Health Care.* London: Chapman and Hall.
Fletcher, L. and Buka, P. (1999) *A Legal Framework for Caring.* London: Macmillan.
Fein, E. and Schneider, S. (1995) *The Rules.* London: Harper Collins Publishers.
Forchuk, C. (1994) The orientation phase of the nurse–client relationship: testing Peplau's theory. *Journal of Advanced Nursing,* 20, 532–537.
Gardener, J. (1992) Presence. Cited in Arnold, E. and Boggs, K. (1995) *Interpersonal Relationships: Professional Communication Skills For Nurses.* London: WB Saunders Company.
Gates, B. (1994) *Advocacy: A Nurses' Guide.* London: Scutari Press.
Gladstein, G. A. (1983) Understanding empathy. Integrating counselling, developmental and social psychology perspectives. *Journal of Counselling Psychology,* 30, 467–482.
Griffin, J. (1997) *Effective Anger Management.* East Sussex: Mind Field Seminars Ltd.
Hadfield-Law, L. (1998) Coping with difficult patients. *UPDATE,* 4th March, 448–452.
Hargie, O., Saunders, C. and Dickson, D. (1994) *Social Skills In Interpersonal Communication,* 3rd edn. London: Routledge.
Hartley, P. (1993) *Interpersonal Communication* London: Routledge.

Hay, L. (1994) *You Can Heal Your Life.* Middlesex: Eden grove.

Health Service Advisory Committee (1987) *Violence To Staff In The Health Care Service.* London: HSAC.

Heron, J. (1990) *Helping The Client: A Creative Practical Guide.* London: SAGE Publications.

Highley, B. L. and Norris, C. M. (1957) When a student dislikes a patient. *American Journal of Nursing,* **9**, 1163

Hobbs, T. (1992) *Experiential Training.* London: Routledge.

Illich, I. (1990) *Limits To Medicine.* London: Penguin Books.

Ingles, T. (1961) Understanding the nurse–patient relationship. *Nursing Outlook,* **9**(11).

Iveson, C. (1994) Solution-focused brief therapy: establishing goals and assessing competence. *British Journal of Occupational Therapy,* **57**(3), 95–98.

Janz *et al.* (1984) Cited in Brimblecombe, N. (1995) Clinical reports. The use of brief therapy as part of the nursing care plan. *Nursing Times,* **91**(35), 34–35.

Jeffers, S. (1992) *Dare to Connect.* London: Piatkus.

Kagan, C. and Evans, J. (1995) *Professional Interpersonal Skills For Nurses.* London: Chapman and Hall.

Keeling, D. I., Price, P. E., Jones, E. and Harding, K. G. (1996) Social support: some pragmatic implications for health care professionals. *Journal of Advanced Nursing,* **23**, 76–81.

Kenrick, K. (1994) Should nurses always tell the truth? *Professional Nurse,* **9**(10), 674–677.

Kiger, A. M. (1995) *Teaching For Health.* Edinburgh: Churchill Livingstone.

Knowles, M. (1986) *Self Directed Learning.* New York: Cambridge.

Kohn, A. (1990) *No Contest: The Case Against Competition.* Boston: Houghton Mifflin Co.

Langford, C. P., Bowsher, J., Maloney, J. P. and Lillis, P. P. (1997) Social support: a conceptual analysis. *Journal of Advanced Nursing,* **25**, 95–100.

Lewin, H. (1969) Cited in Dainow, S. and Bailey, C. (1992) *Developing Skills With People.* London: John Wiley & Sons.

Ley, P. (1989) Improving patients' understanding, recall, satisfaction and compliance. In: *Health Psychology* (Broome, A., ed). London: Chapman and Hall.

Lorig, K. (1992) *Patient Education: a Practical Approach.* St Louis, MO: Mosby Year Book.

Luker, K. A. and Waterworth, S. (1990) Reluctant collaborators: Do patients want to be involved in decisions concerning care? *Journal of Advanced Nursing,* **15**(8), 971–976.

MacGregor, F. C. (1960) *Social Science in Nursing: Application for the Improvement of Patient Care.* New York: Russell Sage Foundation.

Maddux, R. B. (1988) *Team Building: An Exercise In Leadership.* London: Kogan Page.

McFarlane, J. K. and Castledine, G. (1982) *A Guide To The Practice Of Nursing Using The Nursing Process.* London: CV Mosby Company.

Mason, T. and Chandley, M. (1999) *Managing Violence and Aggression.* Edinburgh: Churchill Livingstone.

Menzies, I. E. P. (1968) *Social Systems As A Defence Against Anxiety.* London: Tavistock Publications.

Miller, R. (1990) *Managing Difficult Patients.* London: Faber and Faber.

Morrison, E. F. (1993) Toward a better understanding of violence in psychiatric settings: debunking the myths. *Archives of Psychiatric Nursing,* **7**, 328–335.

Morse, J. (1991) Negotiating commitment and involvement in the nurse–patient relationship. *Journal of Advanced Nursing,* **16**, 455–468.

Neades, B. (1994) How to handle aggression. *Emergency Nurse,* **2**, 21–24.

Nelson-Jones, R. (1991) *Effective Thinking Skills.* London: Cassell.

Nelson-Jones, R. (1993) *You Can Help.* London: Cassell.

Nelson-Jones, R (1994) *Practical Counselling And Helping Skills,* 3rd edn. London: Cassell.

Newell, R. (1994) *Interviewing Skills For Nurses And Other Health Care Professionals.* London: Routledge.

Niven, N. (1995) *Health Psychology: An Introduction For Nurses And Other Health Care Professionals,* 2nd edn. Edinburgh: Churchill Livingstone.

Nolan, J. and Nolan, M. (1997) Self directed and student centred learning in nurse education 2. *British Journal of Nursing,* **6**(2), 103–107.

Norbeck, J. S. (1988) Social support. In: *Annual Review Of Nursing Research* (Fitzpatrick, J. J., Taunton, R. L. and Benoliel, J. Q., eds). New York: Springer.

Ogden, J. (1998) *Health Psychology: A Textbook.* Milton Keynes: Open University Press.

Ogilvie, A. (1980) Sources and levels of noise on the ward at night. *Nursing Times.* July 31, 1363–1366.

Orem, D. (1980) *Nursing: Concepts of Practice,* 4th edn. St Louis: Mosby.

Palmer, A., Burns, S. and Bulman, C. (1994) *Reflective Practice in Nursing.* London: Blackwell Science.

Parsons, T. (1964) *Social Structure and Personality.* New York: The Free Press of Glencoe.

Peel, M. (1995) *Improving Your Communication Skills,* 2nd edn. London: Kogan Page.

Peplau, H. (1952) *Interpersonal Relationships In Nursing.* New York: GP Putman.

Peplau, H. E. (1994) Psychiatric Mental Health Nursing: challenge and change. *Journal of Psychiatric and Mental Health Nursing,* **1**, 3–7.

Persaud, R. (1997) *This Morning Programme.* ITV Television.

Peterson, D. I. (1967) Developing the difficult patients. *American Journal of Nursing.* p. 522. Cited in Stockwell, F. (1984) *The Unpopular Patient.* London: Croom Helm.

Poster, E. and Ryan, J. (1993) At risk of assault. *Nursing Times,* **89**, 30–32.

Powell, J. (1975) *Why am I afraid to tell you who I am?* London: Fontana.

Powell, T. J. and Enright, S. J. (1993) *Anxiety and Stress Management.* London: Routledge.

Reece, I. and Walker, S. (1997) *A Practical Guide To Teaching Training and Learning,* 2nd edn. Sunderland: Business Education Publishers Limited.

Ritvo, M. (1963) Who are the good and bad patients? *Modern Hospital,* **100**(6), 79.

Rodwell, C. M. (1996) An analysis of the concept of empowerment. *Journal Of Advanced Nursing,* **23**(2), 305–313.

Rogers, A., Pilgrim, D. and Lacey, R. (1993) *Experiencing Psychiatry: Users Views of Services.* London: Macmillan/MIND Publications.

Rogers, C. (1980) *A Way Of Being.* Boston: Houghton Mifflin.

Royal College of Psychiatrists (1998) *Management of Imminent Violence.* Occasional Paper OP41. London: Gaskell Royal College of Psychiatrists.

Salvage, J. (1990) The theory and practice of the 'new nursing'. Occasional paper. *Nursing Times,* **24** January, pp. 42–45.

Schwartz, D. R. (1958) Unco-operative patients? *American Journal of Nursing,* 75.

Severtsen, B. M. (1990) Therapeutic communication demystified. *Journal of Nursing Education,* **29**(1), 190–192.

Shulka, R. K. (1988) Structure v people in primary nursing: an enquiry. *Nursing Research,* **30**(4), 236–241.

Siann, G. (1985) *Accounting for Aggression*. London: Allen and Unwin.

Skinner, R. and Cleese, J. (1995) *Families and How To Survive Them*. London: Cedar.

Skodol, A. E. and Karasu, T. B. (1980) Toward hospitalisation criteria for violent patients. *Comprehensive Psychiatry*, **21**, 162–166.

Slevin, E. (1995) A concept analysis of, and proposed new term for, challenging behaviour. *Journal of Advanced Nursing*, **21**, 928–934.

Smith, M. E. and Hart, G. (1994) Nurses' responses to patient anger; from disconnecting to connecting. *Journal of Advanced Nursing*, **20**, 643–651.

Stewart, W. (1993) *An A-Z of Counselling Theory And Practice*. London: Chapman and Hall.

Stockwell, F. (1984) *The Unpopular Patient*. London: Croom Helm.

Sundeen, S. J., Stuart, G. W., Rankin, E. A. D. and Cohen, S. A. (1994) *Nurse–Client Interaction*, 5th edn. London: Mosby.

Tschudin, V. (1993) *Counselling*. London: Baillière Tindall.

Turnbull, J. and Patterson, B. (1999) *Aggression and Violence: Approaches To Effective Management*. London: Macmillan.

United Kingdom Central Council for Nursing, Midwifery and Health Visiting. (1992) *Code of Professional Conduct*. London: UKCC.

United Kingdom Central Council (1996) *Guidelines for Professional Practice*. London: UKCC.

Walsh, M. and Ford, P. (1992) *Nursing Rituals*. Oxford: Butterworth-Heinemann.

Williams, S. (1991) Factors which influence how nurses communicate with cancer patients. *Journal of Advanced Nursing*, **16**, 677–688.

Wright, S. (1990) *Building and Using a Nursing Model of Nursing*, 2nd edn. London: Edward Arnold.

Wykes, T. (1994) *Violence and Health Care Professionals*. London: Chapman and Hall.

Index